Merr̄—

My Card Blen

You + y ours.

In Chit.

Dr. Mll

God's Diet

by
Dr. Neal R. Schiesske

ISBN 0-7414-0629-2

Published by:

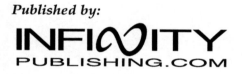

Infinity Publishing.com
519 West Lancaster Avenue
Haverford, PA 19041-1413
Info@buybooksontheweb.com
www.buybooksontheweb.com
Toll-free (877) BUY BOOK
Local Phone (610) 520-2500
Fax (610) 519-0261

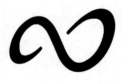

Printed in the United States of America

Printed on Recycled Paper

Published April, 2001

TABLE OF CONTENTS

*This book is dedicated to my
Lord and Savior Jesus Christ who
saved me from death twice, once
spiritually and once physically. Also
to my loving wife Rosa who has been
with me and literally carried me in my
sickness and loved me in health. Also to
my loving children Maria, Veronica,
Joshua, Neal Jr. and Garry.*

INTRODUCTION

In my travels, I have seen many people, in many churches, with many questions. I watched a Church minister on television the other day telling all who were listening how the days of miracles have past. How God no longer performs healings as he did in the Bible. He went on and on about how miracles are no longer needed, now that we all know the truth about Jesus Christ and how he came as the Savior of mankind. I then, as I do now, feel a since of pity for this man, who himself, had the distinctive red face, and difficulty breathing of one who suffers not only of high blood pressure, and high cholesterol, but borderline obesity. My spirit mourned as I watched this man who was himself blinded of the wonderful healing power of Jesus Christ, and at the same time leading his own congregation down the same path. I could picture his congregation as I listened to him. The persons of aging, probably stiff from arthritis and much in the same condition as he, sitting in each row of this man's church every Sunday in pain and agony. And the sad part is, much of the pain and suffering was caused at their own hand, and yet they blame it on the enemy, or accept it as part of old age, or simply part of life.

This book is to enlighten Christians how to take their health into their own hands. It is to show them that the word of God has given a clear and distinctive road to follow, in order to perform this duty. Yes, I said duty! I will show you where it is not only a duty, but a commandment of God, for you to eat correctly and take care of yourself. I will also show you that it is SIN not to carry out this duty. SIN is SIN, to murder, to commit adultery, or to disregard the word of God, it is still SIN.

Therefore, I warn you now! You are responsible for

what you know. And the knowledge in the Bible which is revealed in this book will give you a great responsibility as a Christian, however, you will reap great reward in health and longevity if you heed God's word and take this responsibility to heart. I will give you much scripture during the course of your reading, I would pray that you would take this scripture and investigate this subject in the word of God. For we are instructed to take no man's word for anything, therefore, dig into the word, research, and discover this wonderful frontier of health and vitality found in the Holy word of God.

It is estimated, that if every American gave up red meat and pork for one year, that more lives would be saved from heart disease, cancer, and diabetes, than all of the traffic accidents in the history of this country since the first vehicle was put on the road. My prayer is that this book would educate Christian men and women in the ways of "God's Diet".

ADVERTISEMENT OR DECEPTION?

"Am I blind or what?"

When Rosa and I were first married, we lived in a nice trailer on top of a mountain in eastern Tennessee. The landscape was beautiful. We had a small stream that we could hear running, right next to our front door. A small farm was across the street, and we could see the livestock next to the small farmhouse as we looked out our kitchen window. Rosa is from Puerto Rico, and did not speak or read English very well at the time. One day Rosa decided that she was going to surprise me with breakfast in bed. I woke up to her Spanish accent saying to me "Papi", wake up Papi". As I woke up, I had a lovely breakfast with buckwheat pancakes, honey, and a cup of coffee. I took a sip of the coffee, and immediately spit it across the room. I know it was vulgar, but it was unintentional, and totally unavoidable, for the coffee tasted like a liquid taken from the California tar pits. My actions hurt Rosa's feelings, and after I ate my breakfast, and spent the morning apologizing and explaining to her, everything was ok. Later that day, I was going over a case file and reading Kent's Repertory of the Homeopathic Materia Medica, and saw Rosa standing by the coffee pot shaking her head as though she was puzzled by something. I walked over to her and said "what's the problem honey"? "The coffee has disappeared" she replied. To simplify the outcome, what happened is that Rosa had bought Maxwell house instant coffee and put it through our automatic drip coffee maker. That is the reason for the coffee grounds disappearing from the filter, and also the reason for the sour tasting cup of coffee.

Many Americans who read and speak perfect English make this mistake daily. Rosa simply saw "coffee" written on the front, and picked up the can without a second thought. Every day at grocery stores across America, people are picking up products based simply on what is written in the largest text on the front of the package or can. Other products are bought, based on assumptions made from television commercials, or newspaper advertisements, or radio advertisements aimed to make the American public do just that very thing, buy without knowing the true product or ingredients within. Within the next 2 years, it is estimated that 1 out of every 2 persons living in America will contract a form of cancer during their lifetime. When I was growing up, "cancer" was the word no one said, it was then what the HIV stigma is today. But I can remember that I did not know anyone who had cancer, and I did not know anyone who knew anyone who had cancer. In the last fifty years, cancer and other diseases have become rampant in this country. Today, in contrast, everyone it seems knows someone with cancer, or have had their lives touched by this disease in some way. The only thing which has changed in the past fifty years is the agriculture practices in this country, and the nutritional habits of the American people.

"You are what you drink?"

Billions of dollars are spent every year by large corporations in research for the sole purpose of finding out what makes the consumer remember a specific product, and how to manipulate the consumer into thinking that a specific product would benefit him in some way. "Coke is it", "You've got a lot to live and Pepsi's got a lot to give", are samples of slogans which almost anyone would recognize. This is one example of what I would call questionable advertisement. Soda companies are just one example of this. Beach scenes in a commercial, or a day in the park, just you, your 22 year old model girlfriend and a can of soda, or a day in the mountains are examples of commercialism dedicated to making you think that drinking a certain product will make all of your cares go away. In fact, almost all brown soda's have in their ingredient list "caramel color". Ever seen this in the ingredient list? Of course you have. What is in fact true, is that this color is a derivative of caramel called "2-Acetyl-4-terahydroxybutylimidazole", " THI" for short. This drug in fact is sold to almost all soda companies as a food coloring, and many baking companies as a color for brownies and other consumables. What the ingredients list does not tell you is that this drug, owned by the Coca-Cola company is patented as an immune system suppressant, and used in hospitals for patients who are having organ transplants in order to suppress the immune system of the patient, thus reducing the chances the patients body rejecting the new organ. The truth is, that you are drinking this immune system suppressant and guess what? You are suppressing your immune system. Many studies indicate a much higher rate of colds, flu, sinus problems, and allergies in brown soda drinkers. In addition, the phosphoric acid content of soda is shown to literally cause a calcium deficiency in those who drink them. Ever seen this information in a commercial? I don't think so! I many times ask myself, If my heavenly father were here, would he drink or eat this product? NOT! I promised you I would keep this book simple so I will. The above mentioned is just an illustration of how the American people are being poisoned without our knowledge. It is not only soda pop, it is growth hormones, steroids, additives, preservatives, and pesticides that make the DDT, which was banned in the 1970's, look like water in comparison. Guess what Christians? These things can store up in the fat cells of us, and our children for more than thirty (30) years, and cause serious physical problems many years in the future. In all honesty, as Christian parents, we have to ask ourselves, is feeding our children these poisons good, integral, and spiritual parental behavior?

In closing this chapter, I hope I have planted a seed in you, which will help you to look closer at the things you buy. In later chapters, I will tell you how to avoid these horrible things that are a large part of the health crisis in this country. In one sentence, advertisement only tells us the enticing things that they want us to hear, when hiding the poisons therein. This reminds me of a verse in the Bible, "**Romans chapter 1:22**, "**Professing themselves wise, they became fools**".

"Everyone's opinion is important!..................at least to one person"
N. Schiesske

God Shortens Man's Longevity!

"Honey he's a doctor he knows what's best!"

To our wonderful country, the United States of America, belongs the title of the most powerful country in the world. We have one of the most sought after medical systems in the free world, yet we have one of the highest mortality rates, and birth defects rates on the entire planet. Why, one may ask then, is our system of medicine so sought after? The answer is not a simple one. Our medical system is wonderful and saves many lives, and science is making breakthrough discoveries daily in the fight against disease and illness, unfortunately, many of the diseases our system finds controls and cures for, are also caused by the same system. The reason I say this is that our medical system concentrates on the healing of disease, and almost never, on the prevention of illness and disease. It is estimated that over eighty percent (80%) of all illness and disease is caused by our nutritional intake, yet our medical doctors have little or no formal training in the field of nutrition. Do we then turn to our nutritionist? Unfortunately, our nutritionist, and nutritional experts, are trained with training materials, much of which is provided by the meat producers, cattle growers, and dairy industries as well as other large conglomerates who look only at one thing, no, not our well being, but their bottom line. Another problem with our medical system is that the focus of most of our physicians is covering up symptoms, and not the cause of the symptoms. For instance, if someone would come to a physician with chest pains, heart burn, diabetes, high blood pressure, or any one of a number of problems, most likely a medication would be given in order to cover up the uncomfortable state of the patient, instead of finding out why the person is having the heartburn, or why the person is having chest pains, high blood pressure, or diabetes. Now, lets look at why the average life expectancy of a Medical Doctor in this country is only 55 years of age, and why we as Americans have such high illness, disease, and death rates.

Before the flood of Noah, the life expectancy of a human being was around one thousand (1000) years of age. For instance, Methuselah live to be 969 years of age, Adam 930, Seth, 912, Enos 905, Cainan 910, and Noah 950 years. But Noah, having to build the ark was proof that God was not happy with the human race. Men lived in horrific sin, and had no rectitude or repentance for their actions. Homosexuality, adultery, sexual defilement of every kind, even bestiality was tumultuous. Finally God had enough, and in **Genesis 6:3** the word of God states **"And the Lord said, My spirit shall not always strive with man, for that he also is flesh: yet his days shall be a hundred and twenty years".** There is no other place in the Bible that reverses this statement made by God in this verse. God is literally saying that he will not put up with the immorality any longer, and one hundred and twenty (120) years is to be the life expectancy of man from that time forward. Why the Lord does this is evident in **verses 5 and 6** which states: **"And God saw that the wickedness of man was great in the earth, and that every imagination of the thoughts of his heart was only evil continually. And it repented the Lord that he had made man on the earth, and it grieved him at his heart".** God is literally heartbroken that man had turned away from him and forgotten him, and he, being a jealous God, not only destroyed all of mankind, saving Noah and his family only, but cutting man's life expectancy by ninety (90%) percent, to one hundred twenty (120) years of age. After the flood this becomes evident by looking at the age of man declining such as Shem living only 500 years, Arphaxad 438, Salah 433, Nahor 148, Abraham 175, Isaac 180, Joseph 110, and Moses 120 years. The only age mentioned for a person in the New Testament is Anna the prophetess. We know according to Luke chapter 2: Vs: 36, that she was married for 7 years, and she was a widower for 84 years, consequently, we know that she was at least 91 years old at her death.

"Daddy, will I live to be 47 like grandpa?"

In our world today, things are much different. We find that the average life expectancy for a human being in this country is approximately 76 years of age. What happened to God's statement back in the book of Genesis? I would answer that by saying nothing at all has happened. There are many civilizations on the earth today who average that same life expectancy, ordinarily 90 to 125 years of age. Russian Caucasians, the Yucatan Indians, the East Indian Todas and the Hunzakuts from Pakistan, usually referred to as the Hunza's all live to be an average of ninety (90) to one hundred and ten (110) years of age, and frequently older. In addition, the citizens of these civilization are not arthritic, have no heart disease, no cancer, no illness, usually a full head of hair, and at the time of death are usually prominent, working, and thriving members of their societies, in contrast the American elderly who are usually in wheel chairs, unable to work, in immense pain, and many times end up in nursing homes at 65 or 70 years of age. Beginning to get the picture? Something is wrong in this country! Some people say that the reason these civilizations live so long is genetic, wrong!. Many traits shared by all of these cultures are now believed to be the primary reason for the longevity of these peoples. Three of these traits that I find most interesting, and worth taking a look into. Firstly, they do not eat meat of any kind. Secondly, they all drink water called "Arctic Milk". This is water that comes from the glaciers in the arctic circle and is clouded with many minerals. In fact, when one boils this water down, you would end up with a quarter or half inch of minerals in the bottom of your glass. Thirdly, all of these civilizations have an average of three bowel movements per day. Lets take a look at the significance of these three traits. The absence of meat in the diet is the first trait shared by these civilizations. What significance would this have? Much! The meat sold in this country is contaminated by chemicals such as growth hormones, anabolic steroids, pesticides, and antibiotics. In fact, it is estimated that approximately eighty five percent (85%) of the pork in this country has pneumonia, serious disease, illness or cancer at the time of slaughter. The reason for this is simple. When small livestock in this country is born, one question arises in the cattle owner. How fast can this animal be grown to slaughter size? In order to achieve this, the cattle are given growth hormones, in order to increase their rate of growth. Commonly, steroid injections are given to these animals, not only to help the growth hormones in the speedy growth, but to aid the animal in the pain of ailments such as arthritis, which frequently occurs due to the synthetically produced growth of the animal. The common diet for these animals is made up of many items put in recycle bins weekly by the American households. Newspaper shredded up, grease and tallow that has been recycled, plastic hay, chemicals, and many more disgusting items. The grain that these animals do get, is usually imported from over seas. This is significant in that countries over seas are allowed to use extremely strong pesticides which have been banned in this country. In fact, the only way it is allowed into this country is because it is labeled "not for human consumption". Isn't it ironic, that it ends up in our systems indirectly anyway. Furthermore, because of all of the chemicals mentioned to you so far finding there way into this animals system, the animal gets illness and disease, therefore making it necessary to inject the animal with daily medications such as antibiotics in order to keep it alive, at least long enough to make it to slaughter. If the animal makes it to the young age of slaughter, it is then shipped to the slaughter house. Because of illnesses common on cattle cars, the cattle are commonly given injections before shipping in order to keep them alive on the trip to the slaughterhouse. Many of the drugs used are detrimental to humans if consumed, in fact, many tens of thousands of pounds of meat have had to be recalled from schools across the United States without our knowledge, after the government found deadly amounts of these drugs in the meat, drugs like "Chloramphenicol". Unfortunately, it has not always been early enough, and many times illness and worse has occurred in our schools after consumption of this meat by our children. In addition, Americans are consuming approximately one hundred and fifty (150%) excess protein than is needed to sustain life, due to a meat and animal based diet.

Excess protein consumption can be attributed to cancer, diabetes, obesity, high blood pressure, arteriosclerosis, atherosclerosis, hemorrhoids, constipation, and many other diseases and illnesses. In contrast, the civilizations who eat the most meats, such as the Eskimos, the Laplanders, the Greenlanders, and the Russian Kurgi tribes have the shortest life expectancies on the planet. Coincidence? We as Christian Americans must open our eyes and see how the enemy has slithered in through the cracks of misleading advertisement and governmental trade practices in order to steal, kill and destroy us. God gave us a free will, let us not destroy our bodies with it. Let us instead be wise to the schemes these practices, and treat God's Temple appropriately.

"Arctic milk, it does a body good!"

The second trait of these long living people is the arctic milk they drink for water. Why is this so significant? In this great country of ours, we are truly blessed to have an abundance of food. We can go to the local grocer any time and pick up a meal for our family. Unfortunately, due to the great population, and the intense haste of a society used to being catered to, it has become necessary to make foods that are quick to prepare, or are already prepared for

5

consumption. We have become so accustomed to having whatever we need whenever we need it, farming practices have reduced the topsoil of this country to almost nothing, and the fertilizer use has become astronomical and common practice in order to meet the growing demand of their product. Unfortunately, the quality of the nutritional value of these products have suffered greatly. Farmers use a common fertilizer call NPK, which is the chemical nomenclature for Nitrogen, Phosphorous, and Potassium. Plants do not create their own vitamins automatically, they derive them from the soil they are planted and grow in, therefore, if the soil only has Potassium, Phosphorous, and Nitrogen, the plants cannot automatically produce Beta-carotene, Iron, B-vitamins, and many more vitamins and minerals which are commonly advertised by the American Dietary Association to contain. I would ask you then, how can we in this country get the proper amounts of vitamins and minerals needed in order to keep us healthy. Definitely not from the food, it just is not there. The only answer can be from external supplementation. Again, I turn back a page and restate that Medical Doctors have no nutritional training, moreover, where is one to find out the proper amounts. The medical community cannot even agree on what the daily amounts of vitamins and minerals should be, so how can the general population possibly know? Study to show yourselves approved! God's word says in **Hosea 4:6 "My people are destroyed for lack of knowledge:".** That is the purpose of this book. To increase your knowledge, and open up spiritual blinders so that God's people might see. I will show you later in this book, a general vitamin and mineral regimen, and some books which will help you learn how to treat God's temple judiciously.

"Beef it's not what's for dinner!"

The third trait these civilizations share are there bowel movements. On a normal day these civilization have two to three bowel movements daily. Usually one for every meal eaten. Why is this so important? Our bodies get all of its nutrition from the contents of our colon. The inner membrane of the colon directly osmosizes the vitamins, minerals, amino acids, and other nutritional needs of our body. If a colon contains putrefied animal products which have been there for two or three days, the only nutrition that is going to be given to the body is decayed flesh. This is why a meat eater will pass gas that smells like a dead skunk. Sounds embarrassing, but it's true. That's because the contents in the colon is literally the same as a dead skunk, a dead dog, or any other form of animal found on the highway in northern Alabama. As I said before, in this country, constipation is rampant due to an excess of protein consumption. Animal products eaten by humans dehydrate the colon, thus staying in the bowel for extended periods, thus causing constipation. The end result of this ultimately resulting in lethargy, excessive illness, hemorrhoids, sleep deprivation, and disease. A woman close to me told me last year that she had an average of one bowel movement every three days. As a result, she took chemical laxatives on a regular basis. Her body had become so accustomed to the chemicals, that the laxatives did not work anymore. I suggested that she try an herb called "Cascara Sagrada". She did, it worked, and as a result, got an energy boost, and generally felt better. In the long run, vitamins and minerals are a necessity, and because it is not available in the general food supply, we must take them in a supplemental form. If the proper vitamins and minerals were consumed in this country, illness and disease would greatly reduce in a matter of weeks. In this book, you will learn in general, what vitamins and minerals needed in general, and how to obtain them, which ones are safe, and which ones can have side effects.

"How now poison cow!"

One last topic that I believe fit's in to this topic of longevity is eggs and dairy products. Because of television shows like "Leave it to Beaver, Andy Griffith, and My Three Sons", Americans have always been misrepresented in the matter of dairy products such as milk, cheese, sour cream, and also eggs. Just as red meat, pork, and even poultry, dairy products and eggs contain chemicals which store up in the fat cells of human beings. In fact, the dairy associations, in current commercials state that the calcium in milk, or the vitamin A and D in milk can help you grow. Ever wonder why the commercials do not say "Milk its what a body needs" anymore? What will shock you is that today, more deaths are caused by osteoporosis than cancer of the cervix and breast combined. What does osteoporosis have to do with it you say? Milk adds to the combined protein consumption of a human being. Excess protein eliminates the bodies ability to absorb calcium, thus creating a calcium deficit in the human body. In addition, milk, and excess protein consumption, acidifies the blood of a human being, much like an acid stomach. When a person has an acid stomach, he usually buys an antacid which contains calcium to neutralize the acid content of his stomach. The body does this very same thing. In order to keep the pH of the blood at a proper level, it literally steals the calcium out of the bones of a human being in order to neutralize the blood content, hence creating again, a calcium deficit. When a prescription drug is picked up from the local pharmacy, it usually has warnings of some form on the bottle. Most of the time it will say, "do not take if breast feeding". The reason for this is to

8

advise mothers that the medication they are taking may be passed on to the breast feeding child through mothers milk. Guess what? Cows are the same way. The pesticides they spray on the backs of the cows in order to keep the flies off of them so that the cows can produce more milk, is passed on through their milk just as it is in humans. Are we really drinking this stuff? The same as beef cattle, dairy cows are pumped full of steroids, growth hormones, antibiotics, and pesticides. If the old saying, "you are what you eat" is true, God help us!

In conclusion of this chapter, the life expectancy of a human being on a proper diet is still one hundred and twenty (120) years of age. God's word is still true, it cannot be proven wrong, and it still applies today. The problem being, that in this country, a perfect diet is impossible, pure food is next to impossible to find, but we are commanded, as you will see in the next chapter, to do what we can.

"He that keepeth his mouth keepeth his life: but he that openeth wide his lips shall have destruction".
Proverbs: 13:3

GOD'S WORD AND YOUR TEMPLE!

"Pull up a chair and dig in!"

How important are meals to God? What kind of a question is that, you may ask? **In Exodus 24:8-11**, Moses, Aaron, Nadab, and Abihu, and seventy of the elders of Israel went with Moses, as instructed by the Lord, in order to have a ***meal*** with God, and to seal the new covenant between God and man. In **Mark 14:24-25**, God ate a ***meal*** with his disciples. This meal is commonly known as the last supper. It was to seal the new covenant between God and man. This was the covenant of grace and mercy, prompted because God sent his only Son, our Lord and Savior Jesus Christ, as a sacrifice for the sins of mankind. In addition, Jesus said in **Matthew 26:29 "But I say unto you, I will not drink henceforth of this fruit of the vine, until that day when I drink it new with you in my Father's Kingdom"**, therefore, once again, during the new covenant, marking our eternal life with our Lord Jesus Christ, there will again be a meal. There must be a reason God used food and meals in order to mark his covenants made with man.

That's the biggest church I've ever seen George!

Lets take a look! In the old covenant, the temple of God was a structure, built by King Solomon. It was a fine building, with walls made of the finest woods, covered by the finest gold in the world. **Exodus 26:1** states: **"Moreover thou shalt make the <u>tabernacle</u> with ten curtains of fine twined linen and blue and purple and scarlet with Cherubims of cunning work shalt thou make them"**. A tabernacle is a building. In this current dispensation, God's temple is our bodies. A flesh structure. In **1st Corinthians 3:16,** it begins: **"Know ye not that ye are the temple of God"?** We can derive from this that God 's current Temple is our

10

human bodies.

The Temple of God in the Old Testament was the earthly habitation of God. **First Kings 6:12-13** states: " **Concerning this house which thou art building. If thou wilt walk in my statutes and execute my judgements, and keep all my commandments to walk in them then will I perform my work with thee which I spake unto David thy father and I will *dwell among the children of Israel* and will not forsake my people".** _We know that God stayed in the Holy of Holies with the Ark of the Covenant, and loved his people Israel. Likewise, in the New Testament, God takes delight in dwelling within his temple, which is the bodies of the believers. What an awesome thought, the God of all creation living in us! The creator of all things big and small. It is almost inconceivable isn't it? Again in **First Corinthians 3:16,** Paul states: " Know ye not that ye are the temple of God, and that the spirit of God **dwelleth in you?** " **Also in chapter 6:9** it states: " What? Know ye not that your body is the *temple* **of the Holy Ghost which is in you, which ye have of God".** These verses clearly state that in the New Testament Temple just as in the Old Testament Temple, God has not changed. He still dwells within the Temple of his people, which are, all who confess Jesus Christ as Lord and Savior. In **Hebrews 13:8,** it states: **"Jesus Christ is the same yesterday, today, and forever".** In this context God dwelled within his Temple during the old dispensation, and now, during the dispensation of grace, he is the same and still dwelleth within his Temple.

"God's gonna get you!"

In ancient times, God was very particular what he put into the temple. Nothing impure could enter the chamber of God or touch the items within. **First Chronicles 13:9-10** states **"And when they came unto the threshingfloor of Chidon, Uzza put forth his hand to hold the are; for the oxen stumbled. And anger of the Lord was kindled**

11

against Uzza, and he smote him, because he put his hand to the ark: and there he died before God". Even though the ark was not inside of the temple when Uzza touched it, this shows how particular God is. He cannot be close to sin. His righteousness will consume all impurities. And since God had appointed Levites to attend to his Temple, and even they had to go through a perplexing cleansing ritual before they could enter to care for the Temple, and also could only touch the rods that stuck through the sides of the ark, therefore, no one but a Levite was allowed to touch anything within. In **First Kings 6:7,** it states that King Solomon did not even let the stones which made up the walls be shaped due to the impurity of the iron in the tools, and the impurities of the sound it would make, consequently, he had the stones made in a different place and then brought to the building site. **First Chronicles 28:12-18, First Kings 6:22,** and **Second Chronicles four 4:7-33** all speak of the purity of the wood, ark, candlesticks, and every thing in the Temple down to the smallest detail, was the purest wood, silver, and gold, made by the finest craftsmen in the world. In keeping with his perfect plan, in God's New Testament Temple, our bodies, God has given us an intricate design of miles of blood vessels, arteries, a wondrous cleansing system consisting of organs such as our kidneys or livers, our lymphatic system, a wondrous organ which controls our sympathetic and parasympathetic nervous systems called our brain, and a structure which is so involved, it will never be understood by man. There is nothing second rate given to us by God, thus, again showing us that he is still the same, and though he commanded that the purest forms of wood and metals were used in the ancient Temple, it could not even compare to the abtruse works of our flesh and bone bodies. In comparison, the Temple of God which Solomon built, is insignificant in the eyes of our Creator stacked up against the wonderful intricate structure called our bodies, which he currently calls his temple. Please understand that you are a complex being, and though the Temple of God is made of our body, soul, and spirit in the image of God, for the purposes of this book, we will mainly focus on our flesh and blood body.

In the ancient Temple, all of the workings inside had to be kept clean, filled, and in working order. For instance, the candlesticks could never go out. They had to be kept full of oil at all times. There could be no tarnish on the gold inside the temple. The sacrifices had to be done perfectly, to the letter, in order for the Temple to operate in the perfect harmony God intended. God does not accept second best. As I mentioned before, the priests had to go through a grinding cleansing ritual before they could enter the Temple. In the book of First and Second Chronicles, Leviticus, and Numbers, we can read about the painstakingly intricate duties the son's of Aaron had to go through daily in order to accept any kind of sacrifice. If any of Aaron's son's performed even one duty wrong or foreign to God, they would suffer his retribution. In **Leviticus chapter 10**, we read of two or Aaron's son's who offered strange incense to the Lord. They were immediately consumed by the fire of God. There are many speculations about what made the incense foreign to God, but the fact remains that the priorities God set forth for his Temple were not exercised perfectly, the consequences of their actions was inescapable.

"Citizens arrest! Citizens arrest!"

God also had guards protecting his Temple, and weapons inside the Temple. **First Kings 11:10-11** it states: **"And to the captains over hundreds did the priest give King David's *spears and shields that were in the temple of the Lord*, and the guard stood every one with *his weapons in his hand round about the King from the right corner* of *the Temple to the left corner of the Temple along by the altar and the Temple"*.** This shows that the King kept his armor, and his weapons in the Temple, and outside the Temple were guards at every entrance. In **First Chronicles**

13

15:23-24 it states that Berechiah and Elkanah, as well as Obed-edom and Jehiah were doorkeepers or guards to the Temple of God. In **Second Chronicles 23:9-10** it states: **"Moreover Jehoiada the priest delivered to the captains of hundreds _spears, and bucklers and shields_ that had _been King David's, which were in the house of God._ And he set all the people, every man having his _weapon_ in his hand, from the _right side of the Temple to the left side of the temple_, by the king round about".** This also shows that weapons, armor, and weapons were kept inside the Temple of God. If any intruder attempted to harm the contents of the Temple, ample cautions were taken for safekeeping, and proper police action.

In our bodies, God's current Temple, again nothing has changed. Just as Aaron's sons were killed for their introducing foreign incense. In our current body, a foreign or unclean offering would be a bacteria or a virus. If these are introduced into our Temple, they are immediately consumed by the immune system God has so meticulously intertwined in his modern dwelling place, our bodies. Whenever a streptococcus bacteria for instance is introduced to our body, if our bodes immune system is in tact, immediately t-cells and white blood cells invade and destroy this intruder, thus keeping God's Temple running in perfect harmony. Just as the Temple of old times had guards and weapons at every door, and weapons inside, so does God's current Temple. We have a body that is so advanced, that every cell is guarded. Muscles are guarded and begin to heal immediately upon injury. If we somehow manage to cut ourselves, immediately coagulants begin to clot in order to keep us from bleeding to death. If we are involved in an accident and bruise ourselves, our body warns us of where the injury is by sending electronic signals to our brain, and our brain in return sets the healing process in motion no matter where the injury or how drastic. Just as in the Old Testament Temple, God's current Temple is but a type and shadow of God's intricate scheme, showing his marvelous plan of creation from beginning to end, and again showing that God remains the same yesterday, today, and forever.

So far, in unveiling God's revelation, we have uncovered marvelous resemblance's in how God created his ancient Temple, and his modern Temple in the same likeness. Lets take a look at what we have found out:

OT TEMPLE	*NT TEMPLE*
1.Was a structure with walls	1. Is a Flesh Structure
2. God's earthly habitation	2. God's earthly Habitation
3. Had only the finest contents in his Temple!	3. Has only the finest contents in his temple!

(God was very particular, however, all of the gold, silver, and fine craftsmanship in Solomon's temple could not even remotely compare with the intricate DNA structures, miles of blood vessels and meticulous workings of his current temple, our bodies)

4. There were weapons inside the OT temple! Also were soldiers Inside his temple!	4. The weapons like our lymph there System blood inside his! Cells, etc. are now the soldiers

(There were guards at every entrance to the temple to immediately overcome any known intruder just as a bacteria or virus invades God's current temple, our body immediately attacks it in a preservation effort!)

Thus far, we see how similar God made the Temple of God build by King Solomon resemble, in type and shadow, Gods Temple built by the death and resurrection of Jesus Christ. Now let's take a look at what happens when sin occurs, and the walls come tumbling down.

"My Temple got chicken pox!"

What happened to the Old Testament Temple when God's people sinned and turned their back on him? In **Second Chronicles 36:5-6,** it states: **"Against him came up Nebuchadnezzar king of Babylon, and bound him in fetters, to carry him to Babylon. Nebuchadnezzar also carried the vessels of the house of the Lord to Babylon and put them in his temple at Babylon".** Also in **First Chronicles 6:15, "And Jehozadak went into _captivity_ when the Lord carried away Judah and Jerusalem by the hand of Nebuchadnezzar".** So we see, what happened when God's people sinned, and turned away from the way they should go. The guards were overtaken, the contents were stolen, the Ark of the Covenant taken from the Temple, and the people of God taken prisoner. Now, what happens in God's new Temple, this flesh and blood temple, if we sin and willingly do what we know not to? First of all, let's narrow down the type of sin the Lord instructed me to point out to his people by looking at his word. **First Corinthians 3:16-17** says: **"Know ye not that ye are the Temple of God, and that the Spirit of God dwelleth in you? If _any man defile the Temple of God, him shall God destroy for the Temple of God is holy which Temple ye are"_.** Yes, God said it, that is the way it is. He tells his people, us, that He will destroy any man that defiles his Temple, for his Spirit lives within us! Again God says in **First Corinthians 6:9 "What? Know ye not that your body is the Temple of the Holy Ghost which is in you, which ye have of God and _ye are not your own"_.** God is telling us here, that we do not belong to ourselves. Our Temple, if we are born again Lovers of Jesus Christ, was submitted to him, for his use, the second we asked Jesus Christ to be our Lord and Savior, therefore, we are not our own. Now, just as in the Old Testament Temple, if we allow our oil to get low, or our insides to degrade in some way, we are doing just what God has commanded us not to. How do we let our oil get low? You may ask. If we eat what we are not suppose to, or do not take the time to find out how to treat our bodies properly and give God's temple what is required, God's temple will begin to decay and break down. Just as God's people became prisoners to King Nebuchadnezzar, our temples become prisoners to insulin, chocolate bars, drugs, fad diets, sickness, illness and disease, allergy shots, arthritis pain, blood pressure medication, radiation and chemotherapy and much more. How does God allow this to happen? Let me ask you a question. What is the only item that God allows the devil to eat or consume? The answer is in **Genesis 3:14, "And the Lord God said unto the serpent, because thou hast done this, thou art cursed above all cattle, and above every beast of the field, upon thy belly shalt thou go and _dust shall thou eat all the days of thy life"_.** So the answer is dust. God allows satan only to eat dust. Now lets look at verse **(19)** of the same chapter, **"In the sweat of thy face shalt thou eat bread till thou return unto the ground for out of it wast thou taken for dust thou art and unto dust shalt thou return".** We folks are made up of dust! We will turn back into dust!, and satan can only eat dust! This is how satan is allowed to sneak in and literally eat our bodies. Yes that's right, we give him open reign to do so. He is a legalist and God gave him the right to do it IF he can see it. What! Listen to this! The devil, however, can only eat dust when he can find dust

17

and he is constantly looking for it. We can see this by looking at **First Peter 5:8** which says " **Be sober, be vigilant; because your adversary the devil, as a roaring lion, walketh about, seeking whom he may devour".** Think about it, why is he searching? **Because, as Christians our flesh is not always visible to him!** What! Yes, we do not always walk in the flesh, therefore, *__he can only eat our flesh when we walk in the flesh__.* Let me give you some scripture to back up what I am saying. **Romans 8:3-13** says **"For what the law could not do, in that it was weak through the flesh God sending his own Son in the likeness of *sinful flesh*, and for sin, *condemned sin in the flesh*: That the righteousness of the law might be fulfilled in us, *__who walk not after the flesh__*, but after the spirit. For they that are after the flesh do mind the things of the flesh; but they that are after the Spirit the things of the Spirit. For to *__be carnally minded is death__*; but to be spiritually minded is life and peace. Because the *__carnal mind is enmity against God__*: for it is not subject to the law of God, neither indeed can be. *__So then they that are in the flesh cannot please God__*. But ye are not in the flesh, but in the Spirit, if so be that the Spirit of God dwell in you. Now if any man have not the Spirit of Christ, he is none of his. And if Christ be in you, the body is dead because of sin; but the Spirit is life because of righteousness. But if the Spirit of him that raised up Jesus from the dead dwell in you, he that raised up Christ from the dead shall also *__quicken your mortal bodies by his Spirit__* that dwelleth in you. Therefore, brethren, *__we are debtors, not to the flesh, to live after the flesh__*. For if ye live after the flesh, ye shall die: bur if ye through the Spirit do mortify the deeds of the body, ye shall live".**

Now, we know that these verses talking about our flesh and blood bodies because it says so when it states "quicken your mortal bodies". What about our mortal bodies? First these verses say that flesh is sinful. I will explain what I believe this to mean in a moment. It goes on

18

to say God condemns sin in the flesh. Then to be carnally minded is enmity or separation from God. Then they that walk in the flesh cannot be pleasing to God. Then, we can overcome bodily temptations if we Love Jesus Christ by his Spirit quickening our mortal bodies. And finally, that we are not debtors to the flesh, and do not have to listen to the cravings of our bodies. This applies to the general concept of this book in a very special way. We as Americans every day are carnally minded. Some have weaknesses for chocolate bars, a craving for the milk chocolate taste, or some have to have a glass of milk with their chocolate chip cookies, some are meat and potato men, and there are many more examples I could give you, all of which are succumbing to the temptations of the body. Let me ask you something. If you had a glass of milk and a glass of water sitting on the counter. You just ate two cookies of your choice and had to wash them down. Knowing that the milk was full of pesticides, growth hormones, steroids, and antibiotics, if you were to ask the spirit man in you and allow the Spirit of God to quicken your mortal body in this situation. Which would you drink? Ask yourself this question, which would Jesus drink, after all, Christian does mean Christ like. In asking you this I can say that if you said you would drink the milk, I believe this would be sin. As I have shown you, this would harm the Temple of God, this would be giving into your body, and you would be knowingly doing this, knowingly harming God's Temple and as I have shown you in scripture, **THIS GIVES THE devil LEGAL RIGHT TO EAT YOUR BODY, IT IS MADE OF DUST, AND HE CAN SEE IT BECAUSE YOU ARE WALKING IN THE FLESH AND SENT UP A RED FLAG TO HIM!**

And guess what, you haven't only given the devil the legal right to make you ill, you have angered God. Remember, in Romans chapter 8 he says that HE will destroy those who destroy his Temple, and what is his Temple? YOU ARE! Please Christians, do not give the

19

devil any more than he has stolen, and if you are suffering from illness and disease, I have good news for you, I am going to show you how to get back all he has stolen from you and more. In simplicity, satan eats dust, flesh is made of dust. When we walk in the flesh, he can eat us. If you were to jump out of a moving airplane without a parachute, and decide that halfway down you did not want to die and asked God to forgive your sins he would do so. You would, however, still hit the ground and still be a greasy spot on the ground and die. God will forgive you of your sin, but you will still have to suffer the consequences of your action. The message I bring literally bring the passage of God in **Romans 6:23** that says **"The wages of sin is death; but the gift of God is life through Jesus Christ our Lord"** to life.

In conclusion, the average life expectancy of man is still what God said it was so many millenium ago, 120 years. One reason for the short life expectancy of the people in this country, including, and even more so, the believers in Jesus Christ, is sin in the form of nutrition. This chapter has shown how we are commanded by God to care for his Temple, how there are great and powerful consequences for not caring for his Temple. Not only do we give a "make me sick free" card to our enemy, but we have to deal with God on this issue as well. There is good news, there is deliverance. In the next chapter, we will see how God's Temple can be redeemed, restored, and the enemy can be stopped in his footsteps, buried on this issue, and sent on his way.

"If I see a Godly trait in a man, I pray and ask God if I have that trait. If not, I pray for God to help me instill that virtue into my life!"
N. Schiesske

GOD'S TEMPLE RESTORED!

"There is deliverance!"

Again, lets look at the Old Testament Temple in **Second Chronicles 36:14-17,** which says *"Moreover all the chief of the priests and the people transgressed very much after all the abominations of the heathen, and polluted the house of the Lord* which he had hallowed in Jerusalem. And the Lord God of their fathers sent to them by *his messengers,* rising up betimes and sending because he had compassion on his people, and on his dwelling place. But *they mocked the messengers* of God, *and despised his words* and misused his prophets until *the wrath of the Lord arose against his people till there was no remedy.* Therefore he brought upon them the King of the Chaldees who slew their young men with the sword in the house of their sanctuary, and had no compassion upon young man or maiden old man or him that stooped for age he gave them all into his hand."* This is saying that it is possible for you to be delivered from your sin, illness and disease. It is also saying God will send you a messenger. I pray that this book will be a messenger to many people on the subject of nutritional healing of the body, God's Temple. When God sent the messengers to his people in this passage, however, they turned their back on the messenger and the result was death to all. God was not a respecter of persons, death came for the young and old. I would say to you. Do not turn your back on the message of this book. If you are suffering from illness and disease, God can set you free, but just like any of God's blessings there are certain prerequisites. If a smoker is healed from smoking, and has even one cigarette, he will lose his healing and begin to smoke again. If an alcoholic is healed from alcohol and has one drink, he will again become addicted to alcohol. Any

21

smoker will tell you that it is much harder to stop smoking once you have stopped once and began again, and any alcoholic will tell you that has stopped drinking and began again, that it is much more difficult to stop the second or third time. Why? God's word says in **Matthew 12:43-45, "When the unclean spirit is gone out of a man, he walketh through dry places, seeking rest, and findeth none. Then he saith, _I will return into my house from whence I came out_; and when he is come, he findeth it empty, swept, and garnished. Then goeth he, and _taketh with himself seven other spirits more wicked than himself_, and they enter in and dwell there: _and the last state of that man is worse than the first_. Even so shall it be also unto this wicked generation"**. These verses give a wonderful explanation of why people lose their healings. I have seen people with high blood pressure, cancer, diabetes or some other form of illness or disease come up Sunday after Sunday in many churches for prayer wondering why God has not healed them, or knowing that they received their healing but in wonder of why they lost it. Others knowing that they received their healings, but convincing themselves that the healing was all in their mind, when all of the time, it was just as it is in God's word. They did not take care of their bodies, the Temple of God, and by doing so, gave free reign to the devil to eat their flesh. Their bodies, because of their sin, began to break down, and become diseased. When they prayed, they received their healings, but just as the verses above stated, they went right back to eating the same way and the consuming the same chemical laden foods which caused the disease to begin with, and just as the smoker and the drinker, the cancer demon, diabetes demon, or whatever other demon came back with seven of his buddies and guess what, you invited him in of your own free will. The questions we have to ask ourselves, do I want to make a clear choice to clean my house, to keep it clean, and put the guards back at my windows and doors, and put the weapons of war back into God's Temple, and live the long, health, and prosperous life God's word promises me I can.

22

Do I want to listen to the messenger God gave me. Do I want to walk in the spirit in every way. Do I want to have God's will in all aspects of my life, including the way I eat.

In **Jeremiah 30:17**, it states "***For I will restore health unto thee*** **and** *I will heal **thee of thy wounds*** **saith the Lord because they called thee an outcast saying this is Zion, whom no man seeketh after.**", and in Jeremiah 33:6 it says "**Behold I will bring it *health and cure* and *I will cure them* and will reveal unto them the abundance of peace and truth.**". God says in these two passages that he will bring health to us. If we only ask God to deliver us from these things he will do so. Now that we know the hidden agenda of the enemy, we can cut him off and receive deliverance. God gives deliverance sometimes immediately upon prayer and anointing as he did with my throat cancer, and sometimes God waits and allows us to use the knowledge he has given us. What I mean is that in many cases I have run against, when people begin to treat Gods Temple appropriately, it will simply heal itself. It is, nonetheless, a remarkable piece of work! In the book of **John 17:7** it says "**As thou hast given him *power over all flesh*, that he should give eternal life to as many as thou hast given him.**". This verse states that God gave his son, our Savior Jesus Christ power over all flesh. Guess what, if Jesus had power over all flesh so do we. Scripture confirms this in **John 14:12** which says "Verily, verily I say unto you, he that believeth on me, the works I do he shall do also; and greater works than these shall he **do; because I go unto my father.**". WOW! This is literally saying that the things that Jesus did we are capable of doing also. In this instance what did Jesus do? He had power over all flesh, and in our instance, it is our own. We have power over all flesh. We do not have to eat that candy bar, we do not have to have that 32oz porterhouse steak. I run into people, especially men, and especially in the southeast United States where men claim to be "meat and taters" men, who say to me, "I gotta have my steak, and I gotta have my taters". When I explain to them some of the consequences of their actions, their reply is usually something like "at least I'll die happy". Then when I ask them, what if you don't die? What if you end up in a terminal care center in a coma where your family has to take care of you for the rest of your life. What if you have to die a slow agonizing death instead of a quick heart attack. They usually dodge the subject and to be honest it's like speaking to a brick wall. We have to cry out to God's people! We need deliverance from the snares of the enemy! In **Second Corinthians 6:16** it says "***And what agreement hath the Temple of God with idols*, for ye are the temple of the living God as God hath said, I will dwell in them and walk in them and I will be their God and they shall be my people.**". Fast food hamburgers, pizza, hot dogs, steaks, and JUNKFOOD is the idols I am describing here. A vast percentage of all advertising, television or otherwise pinpoints man's weakness and that is food. The enticing words describes the smells, taste, and seasonings of foods with words such as succulent, or lucious, or tender and juicy, and guess what? We are hooked! Food has become an idol in the Country. Please Christians cry out to God for deliverance. In **Second Samuel 22:7** it says **"In my distress I called upon the lord and cried to my God and he did hear my voice out of his Temple and my cry did enter into his ears."** God hears us when we cry out for deliverance. He listens to us when we realize our sin and cry out for his mercy and forgiveness. And guess what? I believe that this next scripture applies specifically to the purpose of this book, I believe that one of the main reasons for this verse is for God to set free his people from nutritional strongholds, from sickness and disease. Not only is this prophecy about the structural temple to be built, but Gods temple, our bodies! **Amos 9:11** says **"In that day will I raise up the tabernacle of David that is fallen and close up the breaches thereof and I will raise up his ruins and I will build it as in the days of old.".** Also in **Ezra 5:14** it states **"And the vessels also of gold and silver of the house of God which Nebuchadnezzar took out of the Temple** that was in Jerusalem and brought them into the temple of Babylon, those did Cyrus the King take out of the temple of Babylon and they were delivered unto one, whose name was Sheshbazzar whom he had mad governor." In other words, God returned all that satan had stolen from the Temple of God. And because he made our flesh and bone temple so strong, if we cry out to him for deliverance and forgiveness, he will restore our fleshly temples from our illness and disease. I will share with you some stories I have seen with miraculous results later in the book. I have literally seen bodies that look to the medical profession to be on the edge of death come back and live long health lives.

"Oh darn! I forgot to take may pills today!"

One more area I want to touch on if you are going to help restore your temple is drugs. Drugs are wonderful when used properly, however, in America we are very overmedicated, primarily due to people thinking that their doctor knows best. In reality, in America medical doctors are wrong approximately 50% of the time on their initial diagnosis. To restate a fact, approximately 80% of all known illness and disease is caused by nutritional factors, and medical doctors have little or absolutely no training in the area of nutrition whatsoever, therefore, what they do is what they are taught to do in medical school, treat the symptoms, usually by prescribing drugs, which always have some side effects, many times these side effects are detrimental and not seen for years down the road. In **Revelation 21:8** it says **"But the fearful and unbelieving and the abominable and murderers and whoremongers and _sorcerers_ and idolaters and all liars shall have their part in the lake which burneth with fire and brimstone which is the second death."** This ties in with the scripture before which states that God will punish those who defile his

Temple, our bodies. In specific, the word sorcerers here is the Greek word ***Pharmacea*** which is the direct word we get pharmacy from. This word is directly remarking to drugs and people who take them. I believe that God is going to punish doctors who blindly give out un-needed drugs and harm God's people. I also believe that God's people who take drugs blindly upon the advice of their doctors are also in real danger. I read a scary article the other day. It seems that according to Ralph Nader, the research he has done states that 52% of the medical doctors in the United States take Psychotropic or mind altering drugs on a weekly basis! Read the scripture, what does it say! It is your responsibility people, do not let the devil in to destroy you body, God's Holy Temple, as Barney Phife used to say, "nip it nip it nip it in the bud." Please do not misinterpret me as being "anti doctor" or a label of that sort, because I sincerely believe in the wonderful science of medicine and owe my life to it. But when we go and buy a book, we pray which one God wants us to read, when we find a home church we pray for God to lead us to the one that suits his will, and in every aspect of our lives if we follow the word and pray without ceasing, we should want God's will in our lives. But, unfortunately, for some reason when Christians pick a doctor, they go to him or her on referral from someone else, or even worse look in the yellow pages, or after having to go to the emergency room, go to the one they refer us to, when in my opinion, this should be a paramount issue in our prayer lives. There are Christian medical doctors who need our financial support, and who pray over their patients, and pray that God's will be done in the lives of their patients. There are Christian doctors who before surgery, pray for God to guide their hands and that the anointing be used in saving their patients life. This is an ultimate responsibility for the Christian, whether they be a husband, wife, father or mother. I also believe that a Christian should make it a priority to ask their medical doctor if they have studied nutrition, because of the importance of this issue.

In conclusion, God will forgive our blindness, our sin. We have been so blind for so long, and took the word of television commercials and had to drink our three glasses of milk daily, and based our entire diet around a meat center. The devil has literally crawled in without us seeing him and killed millions of bodies of Christians. Now his messenger has been sent. Remember in ***Second Chronicles 36 where it said "and there was no remedy"?*** We now do not have to face those consequences of our willful and ignorant sin, we should cry out for deliverance, and God is faithful and just to deliver us from our shortcomings. Just as he restored the Temple of God from Nebuchadnezzar, and just as he will restore it again to Israel, he will restore his new testament temple. The born again believers of Jesus Christ. Isn't that great news!

If I see an ungodly trait in a man. I pray and ask God to let me see if I have it in me. If I do, I pray for God to help me remove the corrupt trait from myself in order to better serve him!
N. Schiesske

DID YOU TAKE YOUR VITAMINS TODAY?

"Martha, which bottle should I pick? HELP!"

Now that we have established, in God's word, that he cares deeply how we eat, and that it is literally sin not to treat our bodies just as what it is, the Temple of God, in which he dwells, lets begin to learn how to do that. In this chapter we are going to look at vitamins. There are literally thousands of bottles of vitamins in every store we walk in. It is a billion dollar a year industry. The truth of the matter is that in this country, because of the ignorance on the subject of Vitamins, most people who take vitamins are urinating them out and at the same time wasting their money. Many times people are doing themselves more harm than good because they took the word of the clerk at the local health food store saying that a particular vitamin was what they needed. Let's clarify this, shall we?

As I explained earlier, in this country it is next to impossible to obtain the vitamins needed for the proper supplementation of the human body through the food sold in our supermarkets. We, therefore, have to get them through external means of supplementation. When I speak to a patient, I generally use a different vitamin regimen for each person. God made us all in his image, but everyone's metabolism, living conditions, stress levels, and exposure to elements or toxic chemicals are all different. For this reason, we all need different measures and dosages of vitamins. As a general rule, when someone asks me when they see me on the street what is a good multivitamin, I first tell them to read the line just above the ingredient list which states how many tablets you will have to take in order to obtain the amounts listed. It will say something like "each two tablets contain", or "each three tablets contain". A good multivitamin should contain the following:

Vitamin A Palmitate   5000IU
Beta Carotene   25000IU
Vitamin E (Mixed Tocopherols) 400IU
Selenium   100mcg
Vitamin C   500Mg
B-Complex   100Mg   of   B-1,B-2,B-3,B-6,choline, Inositol, and PABA
100Mcg of folic acid, B-12, and biotin

You can usually get all of the above vitamins in a single capsule, or a supplement that requires two capsules. A good mineral tablet I recommend should contain the following:

Calcium   800Mg
Magnesium   400Mg
Potassium   100Mg
Zinc from zinc Picolinate   25Mg
Zinc from zinc Histidinate   25Mg
Manganese   10Mg
Copper   2Mg
Iodine   150Mcg
Chromium   200Mcg

(In addition to this I personally take 1oz of colloidal minerals daily)

This is a good general vitamin and mineral supplement that unless you have allergies to a certain vitamin, should work for just about anyone wanting just a good daily multivitamin and mineral. As always, I am required you tell you to check with your physician or healthcare professional before beginning any kind of vitamin or mineral regimen. If you have a Naturopathic Physician near you, please call him or her and they will be glad to see you and personalize a plan just for your specific needs.

Overdose on Vitamins? No way Dude!

As always, there will be people who go outrageously wild and take much too much of one or more vitamins or minerals. Let me take this opportunity to advise you that too much of anything except for God, can be harmful. This includes vitamins and minerals. Where as vitamins and minerals can be used by someone with knowledge of these things as a healing tool, it can also be used by someone without knowledge of these things, to kill themselves. I would like to name some of the most widely misused vitamins and point out their side effects. The first of these would be Niacin. Niacin is recommended widely by people to treat anxiety or depression, circulatory problems, high triglycerides and/or cholesterol, and it does work for some people. There are two problems with this thought. The first is that Niacinamide or time release Niacin will treat these symptoms on some people with little or no side effects. There have been reported with niacin side effects such as temporary flushing, which turns your face red and sometimes makes you itch. Sometimes niacin can cause duodenal or gastric problems or aggravate a pre-existing stomach problem. If you are taking niacin, however, take it after a meal, this will lessen these effects. There is no known toxicity to this vitamin, however, high dosages such as 2000 Mg daily have been shown to have adverse effects on the liver. The good news is that if this is happening to you, if you stop taking the niacin, the negative liver effects will usually reverse. The second vitamin I want to mention is Vitamin A Palmitate. This vitamin can be extremely toxic. Vitamin A Palmitate naturally occurs in fish liver oil and is fat soluble and stored in the liver. For this reason, it can be very harmful in large amounts. Though there have been some reports of 50,000 IU of this vitamin to cause toxicity, it is rare, with the exception of infants who can have toxic effects with as little as 15000 IU. Some signs of toxicity are fatigue, headache, vertigo, nausea, uncoordination, and body hair loss. All of these symptoms are reversible when supplementation is stopped. Just like Niacinamide, there is a substitute for vitamin A. This is beta-carotene. Beta-carotene, turns into vitamin A in your body, and the remainder is sent to your body for use as an antioxidant, and a pressure reliever for persons with eye trouble. Some people have a problem with Beta-carotene in that it will sometimes make your skin turn a little orange. This is called carotenemia, and it will disappear when you back off from the dosage you are taking. Vitamin D toxicity may be fatal, and unlike the previous vitamins, irreversible. Some studies say that 1000 IU daily of vitamin D appears to be safe, however, there is not agreement on this. When taken properly, vitamin D can be used to battle Osteoporosis and/or high blood pressure. When being used for this reason, the dosage is usually 400-600 IU daily. The symptoms of toxicity of this vitamin are loss of appetite, headache, diarrhea, fatigue, nausea, and soft tissue calcification in the kidneys, bones, and lungs. Vitamin E is one of my favorite vitamins. Most vitamins, however, use only one form Tocopherol, when there are four available, alpha, beta, delta, and gamma Tocopherol. This is the reason for the (mixed Tocopherols) in the ingredients recommendations above. Vitamin E has been found helpful in treating a variety of illnesses including Cancer, Cardiovascular disease, PMS, hot flashes, Poor circulation, healing of wounds, skin illness and disease, and aging. Some adverse side effects may occur, but usually in doses very high, well over 1200 IU daily. Symptoms of toxicity include nausea, flatulence, headache, heart palpitations, fainting, and diarrhea. These are reversible when dosage is decreased. And finally, Magnesium needs to be looked at. Magnesium is known to have no toxicity to most people, unless very high dosages are taken. Dosages in excess of 3000 Mg daily. I can't think of any reason anyone would want to take this much magnesium, however, I though it worth mentioning since the main symptom of toxicity is kidney failure. Please, see a HealthCare professional before beginning any sort of vitamin plan, as you can see, if you do not, it can cost you your life. Be wise! What's good for the goose is not always good for the gander!

The general regimen of multivitamin or multimineral which I mentioned above would be good for a healthy individual on a daily basis, unfortunately, there are many people that are not heatlhy, which is the whole premise for this book. I will mention some cases in which I have recommended different things for different people. Again, I am not advising you to take any particular regimen. You must see a HealthCare professional for that, preferably a Christian Physician with nutritional training, or a Christian Naturopathic Physician. I am just sharing with you some of the past patients I have had, and the vitamin regimen I recommended for them.

"Some of my cases!"

Lets begin with me. Before God healed me of my throat cancer, specifically squamous cell carcinoma and lymphoma. When I was diagnosed, the tumor had reached into my lower and upper jaw, into the origin point of my tongue, and into two lymphnodes in my neck. It was completely inoperable. I refused chemotherapy, but agreed to radiotherapy. I was scheduled for 42 treatments. After the fourth it had completely disappeared. Yes, it was miraculous! This story I will tell you later, but I was preparing my body for radiation treatments, and building my immune system. My goal was to eliminate any side effects from the radiation which I did. I had no nausea, and no hair loss. You will see a supplement called NSC24. This is a wonderful supplement which you can receive literature by calling 1-888-24-NSC24 and asking them for literature. You will also see a supplement called Vitamin B-17. Most medical doctors do not even know that a Vitamin B-17 exists. It is literally unavailable in the American diet, but in civilizations where cancer is non-existent, it is one of the main nutritional sources. You can get information on this Vitamin by calling 1-800-424-1459 or 305-362-3821, or writing to FNI Miami Lakes Dr., Miami, Fl 33014-6997. Anyway, my regimen was as follows:

Beta Carotene	25000IU 3x daily
Vitamin E (mixed Tocopherols)	400IU 3x daily
Vitamin C	2500Mg daily

(To get the proper dosage for yourself of vitamin C, take 500Mg in the morning and 500Mg in the evening. Add one 500Mg tablet in the morning and one 500mg tablet in the evening. When your stool becomes a little watery, then you need to regress to the previous day's dosage. This will be the amount of vitamin C your body needs daily. It is different for each and every individual.)

Selenium	60Mcg 3x daily
GLA	500Mg 3x daily
EPA	1000Mg 3x daily
NSC24	2 capsules 3x daily
B-17 caplets	5 caplets 3x daily
B-17 injectable	1 2x daily
Calcium	1000Mg 3x daily
Magnesium	500Mg 3x daily
Potassium	100Mg daily
Chromium Picolinate	200Mcg Daily
Chromium GTF	200Mcg daily
Colloidal Minerals	1 Oz daily

This is the vitamin regimen I did. Please remember that though this looks like a lot of capsules, much of this comes in one capsule. I do not recommend you take injectable B-17 unless you have a HealthCare professional to administer it under the supervision of your primary physician. I also had an herb regimen, which will be talked about in the next chapter of this book.

The next Vitamin regimen I will show you is one I gave to a patient of mine who was a diabetic. This person was named George. When I met George, he had only one leg. George weighed only about 140 lbs. His family came to me to see if there was anything I could do. I contacted his surgeon, whom I became very close friends with and am still very close to this day. A nurse had to come to George's house daily to change the dressing on the amputated leg, which was taken due to diabetes related poor circulation. They could not seem to get the sore from the amputation to heal. The surgeon told me if I could help, he would be most appreciative, because it was out of his hands. I got to know George and his family. Went to their house and observed his daily habits. Especially his nutritional habits. I made George out a plan with Vitamins and Herbs, and a nutritional guideline which was extensive. I then made a tincture out of black walnut husks and put it on his amputated leg, which began extensive healing in just a few days. The nurse was astonished. The immediate result was good, we were able to get George almost completely insulin free in just six weeks, from his program. We saved his other leg, and three of his toes, and they only had to remove two of his toes instead of his whole leg. His family was very happy. The longterm result was not so good. The enemy got hold of George's mind, and George became very depressed. He varied from my program and began to eat as he did before. The devil whispered to him that he was less than a man because he had only one leg. George eventually stopped taking the recommended vitamins and Herbs. After a few months, he had to start taking his insulin again, they had to remove his leg, and George eventually died. What a liar satan is! This was a battle and war we had won and it was stolen away. The vitamin part of George's program that did him so well is as follows:

Beta Carotene	25000IU 3x daily
Vitamin E	400IU 3x daily
Vitamin C	1500Mg daily
Selenium	60Mcg 3x daily
Calcium	500Mg 2x daily
Magnesium	250Mg 2x daily
Chromium GTF	200Mcg 3x daily
B-Complex	100's 3x daily
GLA	500Mg 3x daily
EPA	1000Mg 3x daily
Colloidal minerals	1 Oz 3x daily

This is the vitamins George took on his diabetes regimen. Keep in mind that the nutritional factors were a great factor in his insulin needs dropping, but the Vitamins taken properly is as much of a factor. When the devil attempts to remind me of George giving up, I simply remind him of all of the victories God has won and how many of God's people I have seen healed with the anointing he has given me of teaching of his people about God's nutrition.

Next, I want to focus on the two problems I incur the most. They are high blood pressure and high cholesterol. Because of the extremely bad diet of America, these two problems are unfortunately, suffered by hundreds of thousands. Due mostly to ignorance on the subject of real nutrition. The following Vitamin regimen is what I recommend to someone who is suffering with high blood pressure or high cholesterol. Please remember, this Vitamin regimen is recommended and will only work when used in harmony with a proper diet, which we will discuss and teach later in this book. It contains the following:

Beta-Carotene	25000IU 2x daily
Vitamin E (mixed Tocopherols)	400IU 2x daily
Vitamin C	500Mg 2x daily
Selenium	60Mcg 2x daily
Calcium	500Mg 2x daily
Magnesium	500Mg 2x daily
Niacinamide	500Mg 2x daily
Colloidal minerals	1Oz 2x daily

This Vitamin regimen along with a proper nutritional and herbal program will 80-90% of the time lower blood pressure to a normal pressure within 6 weeks, if a person follows it to the letter. This Vitamin regimen when followed with an extensive herbal and nutritional program will immediately lower triglycerides and within a couple of weeks lower cholesterol. I have seen triglycerides go from 800 to 100 in as little as two weeks. Keep in mind, however, that the nutritional program I give to people is very extensive and not easy to follow at first. But when people are serious about getting God's temple into shape, they can learn and become accustomed to a new lifestyle. I usually put persons with these illnesses on a six week extensive cleansing diet, and then teach them the lifestyle nutritional changes needed in order to keep God's Temple clean.

One more Vitamin regimen I would like to go over would be for women only. It specifically targets menopausal problems such as cramps, PMS, post menstrual problems, irregular menstrual periods, menopause, and all female problems connected with menstruation, each of which I'm sure all of the female persuasion thank Eve for daily.

Beta-Carotene	25000IU 2x daily
Vitamin A Palmitate	5000IU 2x daily
B-Complex	100Mg 3x daily
Vitamin C	500Mg plus 2500Mg With bioflavanoids
Vitamin D	400IU
Vitamin E	400IU 2x daily
Calcium Citrate	500Mg 2x daily
Magnesium	250Mg 2x daily
EPA	500Mg 3x daily
GLA	1000Mg 3x daily
Chromium GTF	200Mcg 2x daily
Manganese	15Mg 1x daily
Selenium	60Mcg 3x daily
Colloidal Minerals	1 oz 2x daily

IF SUFFERING WITH CARPAL TUNNEL

SYNDROME, USE THIS SAME REGIMEN BUT ADD B-6 100MG 2X DAILY IN ADDITION TO THE B-COMPLEX. ALSO, INSTEAD OF TAKING THE B-COMPLEX 2X DAILY, TAKE IT 3X DAILY.

The above Vitamin regimens is meant to show you how different people can be. In order to devise a Vitamin program for someone, I have to see if they are exposed to air pollution, chemicals, and see the stress levels they are under. Sometimes a family history can be a big factor. And of course, another large factor I have to look at is the pharmaceuticals they are currently taking. There are a few that can cause reactions to vitamins. This is another very important reason you should not take the word of the counter person at the health food store. I would also like to recommend that if you do decide to change your Vitamin program, please look for Vitamins that are plant derivative, and minerals that are naturally derived. Man's synthetics will never improve on what God gave us in nature, and synthetic Vitamins and minerals never absorb, and never have as good of an effect as the natural derived ones. Some Vitamins if synthetic would have to be given in twice the dosage in order to obtain the same absorption levels as natural Vitamins and Minerals.

In conclusion, I can not mention enough, it is important that you seek out a professional, hopefully Christian HealthCare professional to help you devise a plan for your particular needs, and also to keep in mind that in itself, a Vitamin regimen is nothing. But when you include, herbs, nutrition, and most importantly prayer, you have a winning combination. There are also many more facets of Natural Health. Some that I use in helping persons are Shiatsu, Reflexology, Iridology, Massage therapy, Jin Shin Do, Lymphatic Drainage, Acupuncture, Acupressure, and many more, however, prayer, Nutrition, Vitamin therapy, Herb therapy are by far the most important. One more thought! When a Christian's relationship to Jesus Christ is in trouble, and his/her home life is not right, or there is unforgiveness in ones life, this is a strong stimulus for physical ailments. Persons who have a strong church support system, and a close relationship with Jesus Christ can by far heal faster, better, and more completely. If you do not know Jesus Christ as your personal Lord and Savior, turn to the end of this book. He is just a prayer away!

__A man who speaks without thinking and a fool are one in the same!__
N. Schiesske

HAVE YOU TAKEN YOUR MINERALS TODAY?

"John, this stuff comes from tree bark, I'm not taking it!"

Just like Vitamins, herbs are not to be taken lightly. Many can harm you if taken in the wrong way. I, however, will not recommend any of these to any of my clients. There are too many herbs God has given us that will do the same thing without any side effects whatsoever. In order to keep things methodical, I will use the same cases in which I used for the Vitamin regimens, only show you the herb recommendations I made in each case.

The first case I stated was my own, which was throat cancer. Squamous Cell Carcinoma, and Lymphoma to be exact. This was a seven centimeter tumor which had it's poison roots into my upper jaw, lower jaw, tongue origin, as well as my neck lymphnodes. The following herbs are what I took along with my nutritional program and Vitamin regimen:

Red Clover   Two capsules 2x daily

Echinacea   Three capsules 3x daily

Paul D'arco (Tea only) One cup 3x daily

(Paul D'arco is one herb I have found that the medicinal qualities are much higher when stimulated by heat, therefore I recommend the tea and not the tablets)

Sea Weed Capsules   Three capsules 3x daily

Valerian/Ladyslipper Three capsules, and one cup tea 30 minutes before bedtime. (Paul D'Arco Tea) This seems like an awful lot to ingest and keep up with, but when you are fighting for your life, it becomes habit after a while.

The next case was good old George, who was a diabetic. The herb program I devised for George was quite simple:

American Ginseng   One cup 3x daily

Chamomile/Peppermint Tea
(Most diabetics can take natural sugar like fructose or honey to sweeten this tea with)

That's it! Isn't that simple. There are several other herbs that are known to help diabetes, but I have found that the nutritional factor and the Vitamin factor is the most important. These other herbs are Huckleberry, dandelion root, some recommend Goldenseal, however, I do not because it is one of those I spoke of earlier which has been known to have side effects on some people. Uva ursa is another one, but to be honest, through the years, I have not seen much help with this herb. American Ginseng is the best and most potent Ginseng in my opinion, and it gives energy, the Chamomile and peppermint I recommended as relaxing agents. I did this because George was a worry wart.

The next case focused on high blood pressure and cholesterol. In these instances I will first say that if your Naturopath or Physician does or knows anyone who does Chelation therapy, please get in touch with this person. Chelation therapy has been around since 1959, and can clear the cholesterol from an artery that is almost completely blocked in just a few weeks. It has kept thousands from going under the knife for heart bypass surgery. The reason the medical profession swept it under the table in the first place is because of the profit margin. There is little money in Chelation Therapy, but literally millions of dollars in a heart bypass. The following is the herb recommendation for high blood pressure and cholesterol:

Cayenne Pepper (Capsicum) (The hottest you can find)	1 capsule 3x daily
Hops/Valerian Root Tea	1 cup three times daily
Suma Tea	1 cup three times Daily

This is the recommendation I give to most of my cases with these problems. But remember, God made us all different. There are many herbs helpful for these problems such as Fennel, Hawthorne berries, Parsley, Barberry, Black Cohosh, and Butcher's broom, and many more. Depending on the person, and their needs, everyone's herb program may be different.

The final case I used in the Vitamin regimen was for women suffering from a host of serious and bothersome problems such as PMS, Menopause, cramps, irregular periods, and a host of other things that females have to put up with. Though there are many herbs used for these things, I have personally seen the following used. My wife only asked me for help after going to several OBGYN doctors, physical therapists, rheumatologists, and general practitioners. I did not even know she was having a problem until it was so bad she was literally in tears much of the time. There was serious PMS pain, her legs and arms were swollen in the high muscular areas and so sore she could not even touch them. She had fluid built up on these area, and lower back aches monthly so bad she had to be bed ridden monthly for two or three days. The following cleared the problem up, and after she changed her diet and finally followed my advice, the problem has never come back. Her medical doctor and OBGYN gave her prescriptions with terrible side effects, but when I offered to show them the results, though they were undeniable, they would not even discuss the subject of herbs with me. I made a capsules out of the following herbs and gave her two three times daily for six weeks:

Black Cohosh, Peppermint, Strawberry leaf, Valerian root, Blessed thistle, Squawvine, and Milk Thistle.

Paul D'arco tea   One cup 3x daily

This is the program I gave to Rosa. As always there are many more things that can be used for these problems such as Kava Kava, cramp bark, red raspberry, Black haw and Rosemary, and as I said before, each person is different and each person may have a different plan, but an herb plan will only work properly when used with a proper Vitamin and Nutritional program.

Also I mentioned Carpal Tunnel Syndrome. The following herbs are recommended for that illness:

Cayenne (hot as you can get it)   One capsule 3x
                                          Daily

St John's wort (liquid only)   One dropper full
                                      3x daily in
                                      4oz water

Ginko Biloba   Two capsules 3x
                      Daily

In conclusion of this chapter, God gave us plants for

a reason. It is not only for beauty, oxygen and food, but for the healing of the nations. I sincerely believe that for every illness and disease God put a plant on this earth for the remedy. There are billions of species not discovered yet, and the same number destroyed by man daily, especially in our rain forest. Most importantly, as in the Vitamin programs, the most important medication of all, and the most potent by far is prayer, faith, and belief in our Lord Jesus Christ as your personal savior. In our next chapter, we will devote some time to nutrition and God's wonderful plan for caring for his temple.

"Wisdom is not attained over night, but over a lifetime of observation, prayer, and mistakes learned from!
N. Schiesske

YOUR RESULTS! YOUR REWARD!

"Honey, will you make the coffee I'm so tired!"

Integrity is a must for someone who is going to undergo radical lifestyle change which will result in long health and vitality. But many people think God does not see them cheat! Let me tell you God is omniscient. He is everywhere, and if you undertake this journey I am going to lay out for you in the next few chapters, God will give you the strength to learn new nutritional habits, and when you do, you will immediately begin to feel more energy, clearer thought processes, regular bowel movements. In fact, the little aches and pains of life you have learned to live with will suddenly disappear without you even realizing it. It is wonderful the benefits and rewards given to us when we decide to obey God.

There are a few things I need to let you know about. If you are going to undergo my six week cleansing diet discussed later on in the book, you will need to be prepared for some withdrawal symptoms we Naturopathic Doctors call a "Healing Crisis". Usually during the end of the second week or the beginning of the third week of the cleansing diet, you may begin to feel lethargic to the extreme extent. I have had patients not even get out of bed. The reason for this condition, simplistically put, is because your body, no longer having to deal with all of the poisons and processed foods being introduced into it, has gone on a literal cleaning rampage. You see when your system is not having to deal with every day junk being put into you system, it is able to begin to clean out all of the stored junk you have put in it your entire life. In other words, your body is stealing all of your energy in order to clean all of the drugs, chemicals, and every other unclean thing it has stored in your fat cells for the past 10, 20 or 30 years. In order to do this, it needs all of the energy it can get. This stage usually last from 7-10 days. Many people give up and say it is just not worth it to feel this way, but many who tap into the Spirit of God see it as a blessing and a lesson learned and God shows them the light at the end of the tunnel.

After this stage, you will come to the energy stage. This has some good attributes and bad. All of a sudden the lethargic stage will be gone and you will have an excess of energy. This happens when your body catches up on it's cleaning duties and is able to allow you to function properly and still keep the cleaning process going. You are not completely cleared out at this point, in fact, it is estimated that to completely clean one's fat cells and body from contamination, it would take one entire month for every year lived. But during this stage, I have had patients call me at 3:00 o'clock in the morning telling me that they cannot sleep, or that they feel like they could run a marathon.

This stage which people usually welcome despite the sudden lack of sleep does not last as long as the lethargy stage. The energy stage usually lasts about 3-5 days. After that you have got it licked. You will be able to concentrate on new and improved ways of making your new diet more fun for you and your family. Remember, this usually occurs if you choose to go on the six week cleansing diet. After the six weeks, you will be able to use the recipes in this book, or make up your own, in order to make your nutritional lifestyle change a fun and pleasant one. Also remember, everyone does not go through the above stages, and when someone does, it is not always as startling as described above, but I felt it necessary to give you a worst base scenario to prepare you just in case.

"The rewards are great!"

In the remainder of this chapter I wanted to tell you of some of the success stories I have seen. Some of them may seem miraculous to you, but God is a miraculous God. These are from my case files in the Alternative Health Clinic, and Natural Health Clinic's in Central and Eastern Kentucky and Tennessee. When I first interview a client, I inform them about God's miraculous power. I then pray with them if they will. I then inform them that I do not make any recommendations on the first day, that after we talk for an hour or an hour and a half, I will then take their case file and pray that evening for God's guidance on the proper recommendations for this particular person. I schedule them for a follow up, usually the next day, or the day after. When they return, I sit down with them, go over in extreme detail the program I think is appropriate for them, go over their shopping habits, eating habits, if I recommend acupuncture, homeopathy, reflexology, lymphatic drainage, but always, a Vitamin, Herb, and Nutritional Regimen. We discuss this and set a beginning date and a goal for the person. The day before the beginning date they will go grocery shopping, and do spring cleaning in their home. They discard the things they are not

allowed to have. These things will be given to you in chapter 8. Then on the morning of the beginning date, I give them a call just to support them and make sure everything is on track. The following cases are from those case files of people that did my recommendations to the letter, thereby receiving the full benefits and rewards.

"Barbara"

Barbara was an English lady of 71 years. She was very proper in her language and mannerism's. When she first came to me, she was very cautious because she had never heard of a Naturopathic Doctor before. She was recommended by a work associate. I was at that time, the Nutritional Director for the Kentucky State Contact Agency for the mentally retarded. When Barbara first came to visit, she and I sat and talked about all of her physical problems. After an extensive talk, I looked over her symptoms. When I looked at her feet, she showed no signs of extreme toxicity. Barbara had been incontinent for over 30 years at that time, and did not give much hope of being helped. She had been wearing adult diapers for many many years, and just wanted to explore all possibilities of being free. Barbara was not a born again Christian, but I pray that I was able to plant some seeds into her heart that will blossom. Barbara was an easy case. Doctors had put her on so many medications through the years she had given up on them. I found that Barbara's diet was on the average very good, and she was somewhat apprehensible about changing it any more. I sent off to Starwest Herbs in California. I have found that they have herbs with very high medicinal value. Rosa and I spent two days mixing and making up capsules for Barbara. After only a four week period had passed, Barbara called and made an appointment. Rosa told me she probably needed some more capsules. I had made plenty and kept them in a freezer just in case. I will never forget the day she drove up. As she walked up the front sidewalk to my office, I saw that she was crying. I was concerned and invited her in. She entered the front door first and I followed only to have her arms immediately around me. In her English accent the words are burned into my mind and spirit, she said; "I'm free, I'm free, I've been wearing those stinking diapers for thirty years and I'm free". Of course I began to cry as well, in fact, I'm crying as I write this for you because of the remembrance in me. This is truly how God works in all endeavors. He sets people free. I gave her the recipe for the capsules, gave her a years supply and occasionally checked on her. The last time I spoke to her, she was still free and doing fine. The reason I included Barbara's story is that without her being having been brought up with good nutritional habits, the herbs given to her probably would not have worked. Diet is paramount in staying healthy.

"Janet"

Janet was the secretary for the State Contact Agency I mentioned before. She first came to me with back pain. She was a wonderful woman, but her stress level was extremely high. The first time she came to my office, she was so uptight she could hardly talk. I had some Lobelia tincture I had made and as we sat and talked, I asked her if she would mind taking just a tablespoon of it every few minutes. She agreed. After about an hour and four tablespoons of lobelia herb, she was so relaxed, she was laughing and telling Rosa and I jokes. I remember that day as very jovial. Janet was a heavy smoker and unwilling to give that up, so I had to work around that. After extensive talking and examination, the Lord told me that the uric acid content in her lower back was excessive, and because bacteria thrive on uric acid and multiply as a result, the muscles in the lower back were inflamed. I have found that kidney strain from processed foods and chemicals especially preservatives are many times responsible for this. Janet was willing to go on my six week cleansing diet. She went through the normal stages, and at the end of the six weeks, not only had her back pain disappeared, but she had lost 15 pounds. We then sat down and taught her how to plan her own nutritional future. The last time I saw her, she was still on her vitamin and herb regimen and had lost a total of 24 pounds. God is wonderful isn't he?

"Crystal"

Crystal is a wonderful memory for me. She was forty-one years old when I first met her. Even though she was a young woman, her appearance was one of a person who had live many years. She was slumped over and had obvious signs of osteoporosis. When I spoke to her, she told me that she was having to quit her job. She said she just couldn't seem to get up in the morning and go to work due to her energy void. She told me that this had been going on for about two years. When I examined her, I found mild curvature of the spine, back totally out of alignment, but something I had not expected. Every trigger point on her body pointed to extreme toxicity. She also had three nerve rings in the iris of her eyes pointing to debilitating stress levels. When I see one nerve ring, it is usually someone not getting along with their boss, or a child getting bad grades in school. When I see two nerve rings, it is usually on the level of someone getting a divorce, or going through an extremely tense episode in their life. When I see three nerve rings, it is usually someone on the brink of tears. It is usually when someone has lost a loved one such as a spouse or child. It was this I saw in Crystal. When I confronted her with it, she admitted that she had been contemplating suicide. I shared the salvation of the Lord Jesus Christ with Crystal, and though she did not receive Christ as her personal savior at that meeting, she later did. Anyway, after two hours of conversation with Crystal, I had found out that she was brought up on a dairy farm. Her job as a child was to hold a hose which sprayed pesticides and spray the pesticides on the backs of the dairy cattle in order to keep the flies off of them. This reduces the stress of the cattle, thus, helping them produce more milk. These pesticides had been stored up in Crystal for more than thirty years and just now taking their toll on her body. After lymphatic drainage, shiatsu, and most importantly, a vitamin, herbal, and extremely strict nutritional program, in about three months Crystal looked like a different human being. Rosa and I still think about her. I would see her every now and then when she would just out of nowhere pop into my office door, give me a quick hug and peck on the cheek to let me know how she was doing, and disappear into the day again. She had literally turned from a diseased, lethargic person on the brink of suicide, to a perky bundle of energy unable to stop. It was as if she was making up for lost time. Praise God for his miracles.

"Anita"

Anita was a secretary for the local Farm Bureau Insurance Company. She was from Columbia and was a fluent Spanish speaking person. She and Rosa got along just fine, although, when they got together, no one could understand a word they were saying. The first time I got a call from Anita, she spoke very softly on the phone. The reason for the soft tone was apparent she was suffering a migraine. As she spoke so softly she introduced herself to me, telling me of a migraine headache she was currently suffering. She said she had suffered from this one for three days. She had been to the emergency room twice and received two shots on two different days that put her to sleep, but upon waking up, still had the migraine. I asked her if she had someone to drive her to my office, and she informed me yes. When she arrived, she had on dark sunglasses to keep the light from her eyes. She slowly walked up the stairs, and I turned off all but the bare necessary light in the house and walked her down the stairs to the exam rooms. I laid her face down on the table and while Rosa got my acupuncture needles and supplies ready, I applied acupuncture on her. While I began Anita's treatment Rosa had two ladies come in and go into the massage room with her. One of them was her appointment and the other a friend that came with the appointment. After I had applied the needles, I administered a sonic machine to two of the acupuncture needles. After a half hour treatment, I removed the needles. Anita got up from the bed, she looked around, removed her glasses, and began to scream at the top of her lungs in Spanish. The two ladies Rosa was with, one half dressed ran out of the massage room, they thought this lady was injured or crazy one of the two. Rosa was just smiling. After moving as far away from Anita as I could, I inquired to Rosa about what she was screaming about. Rosa informed me she was screaming "Praise God, Praise God, I have been set free, three years and I am free". She went on and on, and after a great while Rosa was able to calm her down, and I saw tears streaming down from her face. This reminded me of Barbara from the first story when she cried. Later, almost completely with changing her diet, we were able to completely eliminate her migraine headaches. The last time I saw her, she had two of the restaurants she frequented making special meals just for her and she had been free for over a year. Praise the name of our Lord Jesus!

"Lynn"

The next story is of Lynn. Lynn was a secretary of a cardiologist. She had suffered from cardiac arrhythmia for many years. When I met her, she could hardly walk across the room without beginning to breathe heavily. She told me that she came to see me after seeing the result of a patient of her bosses had recovered from an illness he could not help her with. She also told me she was afraid to tell her boss because he thought Natural Health was voodoo medicine. So I set her at ease by letting her know I would not tell her boss. Lynn was an easy case. With vitamins and a nutritional program change, she was able not only to rid herself of her problem, but she began to hike in the mountains on the weekends and bike ride. As most Americans do, she ate badly. Her problem was simply her bodies way of saying HELP! It took about three months to rid her of her problem, but God provided a way. Isn't it great how God made us!

"Wilda"

My next story is about the person who ignited Lynn's interest. Her name was Wilda. I had never heard that name before, but she was an extremely sweet lady who loved Jesus. Wilda was about 75 years of age. When her daughter brought her to see me she advised me that she had just been released from the hospital. She was suffering from heart congestion, and had been for some time. She told me that her heart was extremely enlarged, and the doctor advised her to stay in the hospital. Her daughter told me that the doctor didn't think the prognosis was good. Wilda told me if she was going to die, she was going to die at home and not at the hospital. I informed Wilda that I was not a Medical Doctor and was not capable of taking care of a heart patient. She insisted I do what I could, so as always, I wrote a letter to her cardiologist, and got no response. I then called his office, and he hung up on me. I prayed for guidance, and told Wilda that her doctor refused to help me in this task. I put her on an extreme cleansing diet, Vitamin and Herb program, and had her buy a juicer. She was instructed to make a vegetable juice cocktail three times daily using twice as much cabbage as any of the vegetables. Cabbage is an extremely strong diuretic. When used properly it not only works better than pharmaceuticals, but there are no side effects. Wilda began to see immediate results. In only four weeks, her doctor told her whatever she was doing to keep doing it. Her daughter told me that the doctor had confidentially told her that he never thought she would make it this long. At her two month checkup, her congestion had completely cleared up, and her heart had gone back to the original size. Later that year, I was in the grocery store parking lot and heard someone screaming from the other side of the parking lot. It was Wilda, she was telling the person she was with, there he is, he saved my life. To my surprise, she ran to greet me, gave me a hug, and we had prayer and thanked our Lord Jesus Christ for life.

The last story I am going to share with you is my own. Last February I noticed an abnormality in my throat which immediately discouraged me. I went to the emergency room at the hospital my wife works at. He set me up with an Ear, Nose and Throat specialist the next day. When I went to see the specialist, he stated that it looked like Squamous cell cancer and a biopsy was needed to confirm his suspicions. The biopsy was scheduled and the results were positive, and confirmed his beliefs. He then sent me to an Oncologist who specializes in throat cancer. He told me of an experimental antibody called C-225. This was not a drug, so I gave him the go ahead. He told me that my

53

chances with this new drug was high, because it blocked the cells in the cancer wall from duplicating. He scheduled me for my first administration that Friday. The next week I was to have it once weekly just before my radiation treatments. I went in for my first administration and was immediately concerned when they set up a cardiac crash cart just in front of me during administration of the intravenous needle. When they began to pump these antibodies in, first I began to itch and broke out with large red spots all over my body. They then injected me with Diphenhydramine in order to counteract the reaction. They continued and I began to black out. They stopped the drainage of the antibodies and I came back to reality. They began the drip of the antibodies again and this time it was like I saw my vision begin to tunnel. I knew I was going night night, and I knew I had to do something because the nurse and doctor was in the other room. I reached over and stopped the drip myself and rang a bell which was next to me. This was the last thing I remember. I then instructed them not to administer any more of the antibodies. The only thing left was radiation, so we scheduled that to begin the next Thursday. During the past month since my diagnosis, I had began to build up my bodies immune system in order for it to withstand radiation if needed. I took the vitamin, herb and nutritional program I outlined for you in the vitamin and herb chapter. The doctor called me in his office the Wednesday before the Thursday I was to begin radiation and told me, in his words: "Your cancer not only goes into your upper and lower jaw and lymphnodes, but it's tentacles have reached into the tissue where your tongue begins, and removal by surgery would be impossible". I thanked him for his candidness, but felt a calmness from the father all of this time. The next day, I went in for my first radiation treatment. Friday, I went in for another. I felt no soreness at that time and thought to myself how easy this was going to be. That Sunday, at church, I went to the front for prayer. My assistant pastor, Darryl Eubanks, came up behind me and prayed for my healing. I felt the power of God strongly. That evening while I was watching the 700 Club, Pat Robinson's son gave a prophesy. When he gave this prophecy, the hairs stood up on the back of my neck, he said: "The person I am speaking to has a growth in his throat, and it is into not only his jaws, but it has it's tentacles into the place where his tongue begins, and it is melting away at this time, God is healing it now"! The exact words of my doctor the Wednesday before. I got down on my knees and claimed that prayer for myself, and thanked God for his mercy and kindness. Monday and Tuesday I went for my 3rd and 4th radiation and Wednesday, I went to my weekly appointment with my doctor. When he came in and looked into my throat, I saw a look that concerned me on his face. All of a sudden he began to jump up and down like a teenager, he called my wife, Rosa, his nurses and everyone he could find to look down my throat. He said "its beautiful!, no I don't mean it's beautiful, but It's beautiful, It's all gone, nothing is there!". I began to cry and looked at Rosa. She knew what I was thinking. God had miraculously healed my throat cancer. In wisdom, I continued my radiation treatment, because, my doctor gave the glory of my healing to the small amount of the antibodies I had received, but I know in my spirit it was many things. Firstly, the power of God. Secondly, the strength of my immune system due to the supplementation God told me to take, and third, but by no means least, the prayer of my friends and loved ones.

The radiation treatments got almost unbearable, and I lost 100 pounds, but God had a purpose. Many good things came from this. After my not being able to take the antibodies, my chances of survival came down considerably. When these things happened to me, my eyes opened, and God revealed unforgiveness in my heart. I repented and prayed for forgiveness, and relationships were healed that had been torn from unforgiveness, and many more good things happened. My wife, children and I became and still are closer than ever. But the most amazing thing was God opening my eyes and letting me know that I needed to get off of my can and do what I was anointed to do.

In conclusion of this chapter, I pray that you would see in these real cases, that God can work many miracles in peoples life. He, however, expects you to do your part and take care of his temple, and allow it to do what he has built it to do, heal itself. I still am very picky about eating what I should, because I will not allow satan to enter into my life in any way or form. When I grocery shop, I pray for God to give me wisdom, when I prepare the meals for my family, I do the same, because I know I am responsible for teaching my own children strong and proper nutritional habits which will ultimately lead to their living long and healthy lives. May God be praised!

"She openeth her mouth with wisdom; and in her tongue is the law of kindness."
Proverbs: 31:26

NATURALLY NUTRITION!

Nutritional Experts! NOT!

It's time to get down to the nitty gritty, life saving subject of nutrition. To begin this chapter, I would like to show you how God made you body to respond to things found in nature in a positive way, and synthetic things made in a laboratory in a negative way. I already touched on this subject in the vitamin section, but now, we will dig in a little deeper to further your understanding on this subject.

I always get a little agitated whenever I am watching one of these medical doctors or so-called nutritional experts on television telling his audience something is good for you, or something is bad for you, and expect us to believe that this is true for one and all. It use to be that they said, for instance, that salt was bad for you. Then they changed it and said Salt was bad for you, only to change again and say it was beneficial to you, and now they are split. Some say it is good for you, and some say it is bad for you. The reason for my agitation is simple. These people are making things much too complicated. They do not understand the concept of organic Vs inorganic. They do not understand that God made man and his body to respond to natural things. In **Genesis 1:29** it states **"And God said, Behold, I have given you every herb bearing seed, which is upon the face of all the earth, and every tree, in the which is the fruit of a tree yielding seed; to you it shall be for meat.".** This means that God originally intended man to be a vegetarian. Please don't get me wrong, I am not trying to turn anyone into a vegetarian, that is between you and God, I only want to state the facts, and God intended for Adam to eat only herbs bearing seed, fruits and nuts from trees, and leaves from trees. In fact, meat was only introduced as a result of sin. The first animal sacrifice was only carried out because of sin in the Garden of Eden. God killed an animal in order to make clothes for Adam and Eve because of their nakedness. Our God is not wasteful, and I'm sure Adam had to eat the meat thereof, even though this is supposition. Ironically, it was right after this sacrifice and I believe meal, which God informed Adam and Eve they would eventually die and turn back into dust. The point I am making is that the human body was originally intended to ingest only natural things.

Four examples I like to enlighten people with are the consumption of Sulfur, Sodium, and Sugar, and Mercury. The first, Sulfur is naturally occurring in many plants such as garlic and onions. It is a wonderful natural antibiotic and antiviral agent. In fact, garlic was so important as a medicine, that it was 1st prize in the first Olympic games in ancient Greece. It was often times killed for in the 19th century. During the black plague of Europe, the only doctors who survived the plague were the ones who ate cloves of garlic every morning before they treated their patients. The most famous of these physicians was Nostradomas. The inorganic form Sulfur is not derived from plants, but manufactured for use in things such as match sticks. Though the chemical consistency is the same for the inorganic and organic forms of sulfur, if one were to scrape off a small portion of the inorganic sulfur from the end of match sticks and ingest it, the results would not be good. One would get a furry coating on his tongue. Perhaps begin to sweat through the pores of the skin an orange substance with an obtrusive odor. And have a headache the size of Texas. This would result of the human body reacting to a synthetic, un-natural substance being introduced to it. In contrast, thousands of milligrams of natural Sulfur in garlic and onions, herbs and spices, are ingested by people all over the world, and none of the side effects normally occur when the naturally obtained sulfur is introduced to the body.

The second substance is Sodium. Sodium is usually found in the form of Sodium Chloride or table salt. The reason for scientists not understanding if salt is good or bad for you is that they do not understand how God made our bodies. Like Sulfur, Sodium is found in almost every fruit and vegetable we eat. We literally ingest thousands of milligrams of sodium daily as Americans. Yet, only when ingesting the inorganic, synthetic form of sodium, such as table salt does the body have side effects. No side effects would be seen if we ate pounds of vegetables with sodium, but if we ingest only a small portion of the inorganic type, (table salt) many of us would find ourselves retaining excess water, and perhaps undergo a rise in our blood pressure. Again, we see how God made our bodies to thrive on the natural things he made for us to eat.

The third substance is sugar. Hundreds of thousands of pounds of table sugar is ingested daily by Americans. It is added to almost everything on the grocery shelf. Next time you go to the grocery store, look at the children's cereal that state that they are part of a nutritious breakfast. Ninety-five percent of the cereal has added sugar and salt. Again lets look at this synthetic product. Table sugar comes from sugar cane, however, it is not in it's original natural form, but processed in a plant. Because of this, the human body seems to have an aversion to this product. For instance, if a diabetic were to eat a tablespoon full of table sugar, he would probably go into sugar shock, or perhaps have a seizure. Why then, are most diabetics able to eat natural occurring sugars like honey, unsulphured molasses, or fructose which is sugar derived from plants. For the same simple reason. The human body only thrives on naturally occurring foods. Isn't that simple?

One final substance I will mention if only to educate you on how a small amount of poison can do a large amount of harm. The substance is Mercury. One (1) mg of Mercury, about 1/5 the weight of a nickel, or the amount used in a thermometer is enough to pollute a twenty (20) acre pond, and kill all of the fish. There is, however, an organic form of this substance that is completely harmless to human beings and the environment alike. Why do we not use it? The answer to this is money! Many foreign nationals mine Mercury, and provide income and employment for their governments. We, by purchasing the products which contain this mined Mercury, are essentially saying that money is more important that human life or the environment.

"John, buy me that diet that I saw on TV!"

This same premise can be seen in many foods, for instance, we hear of all of these fad diets concerning carbohydrates and the abstaining thereof. This concept has men and women all over the world missing many of the wonderful foods God has put on the earth for us because scientists say it is making the American people ill and obese. Well, they are partly correct, it is making the American people ill and obese, however, again they do not understand the concept of God's creation. This concept is not new to me, I have been practicing it in a form for years. Let me explain. When people eat the processed forms of these foods such as spaghetti noodles, white rice, macaroni, or any other processed white pasta, white rice, white flour, or sugar, they are eating an inorganic products which has been processed. Men processed these items because they thought they could improve on God. That's why you will read "enriched" in the ingredients column, unfortunately, it is causing kidney failure, liver problems, elimination problems, blood problems and a hosts of illnesses and diseases caused by the human body being broken down year after year of being forced to ingest these inorganic things. When I recommend a nutritional program for someone, besides prayer, the first thing I teach people is to eat the organic forms of these products. THATS RIGHT! You do not have to go without.

When you give God's Temple the natural forms of these things your body will recover. Just as in the previous examples of sulfur, sugar, and sodium, there are organic substitutes for flour, white rice, pasta and just about every other thing. For instance, instead of white rice which is not only processed, but many manufacturers use polish which in itself is a cancer causing agent, use whole grain rice made from whole wheat, barley, spinach or another substance. Instead of white flour use soy flour, whole wheat flour, or barley flour. Instead of spaghetti noodles, used spinach, whole wheat, or any of a number of different kinds of noodles not made from enriched flour. You get the picture. The following is a list of the most frequently used products I have found to help my clients in their shopping and their substitutions:

Spaghetti & other noodles	Whole grain noodles, Spinach, soy, whole Wheat noodles
Sugar	honey, fructose (diabetic Section)
Milk	Vanilla soy milk (Haines Tastes best)
Flour	Whole wheat or soy flour
Eggs	Egg substitute
Salt	McCormick's 17 seasonings, Mr. Dash
Cheese	Soy Cheese (grocer, health food store)
Hamburgers	Morning star meatless

	products
Hot Dogs	Morning star meatless products
Rice	Whole wheat or Brown rice
Vegetables	Frozen, or no salt canned (Prefer frozen)

If one eats the natural forms of these foods instead of the processed forms, he can expect the same result as if he had completely given up carbohydrates altogether, in most cases. In other words, you do not have to go without to get results, just treat your body with natural foods. That's what it was made to run most efficiently on.

"That came from a cow you know!"

In the next chapter I will be teaching you how to make your favorite meals using natural products, however, there are a few things I must substitute in order to obtain a product which I think suitable for God's temple. By suitable, I mean a product God's temple will not react to because of it's being processed and synthetically produced. Some of these products have chemicals in them such as "I can't believe it's not butter spray". The reason I will include products like these is that most American's get very frustrated very fast when it comes to taste, and in order to make the food taste appealing, it is necessary. I will put an asterisk * by these products. The asterisk will represent my preference to be that this product not be used, but if it is absolutely necessary for you to use something, this is the most appropriate.

Many products are so bad, I will recommend that you never

use them, such as dairy products, eggs, processed foods, sugar, salt, butter etc. I will, however, provide appropriate substitutes. Most of the substitutes I will use are available in your local supermarket, including soy bean meat substitutes, but if you are unable to find them there, please check your local health food store.

In conclusion of this chapter, I hope that you understand the simplicity of God's original plan. He planned our diet to be simple, he created our bodies to live on simple things, an though he made our defenses tough, just like the Old Testament Temple which was finally torn down by the Romans, if God's new temple, which is his people is fed badly day after day, year after year, it too will break down and fall down. This book is focused on teaching you how to avoid this and become the temple guard God directed you to be.

"Pride is one poison that will never injure one to swallow!
N. Schiesske

THE DIET AND RECIPE'S

First, I want to show you my six week cleansing diet, vitamin and herb program. As I have stated many times in this book, this program is a general program and would suit the average person. Below is a list of absolute NO's for the six week diet. (read the ingredients list to see what you have bought, if sugar is on the list NO!)

Salt

Dairy products (Including milk, cheese, sour cream, or anything with dairy products added)

Eggs (not even free range eggs, and no egg substitutes)

Red Meat

Pork

Processed pasta or noodles (White or enriched)

White rice

Coffee

Soda's

Tea

Butter

White potatoes

corn

Salt free substitute (containing potassium Chloride)I hope I have not discouraged you, but it is important for the initial six weeks. The good news is that I have some recipe's for you to follow.

Please remember, when I say read the ingredients list, I do not mean the ingredients chart. The chart may say sodium or sugar on it, but when you look on the ingredients list, salt or sugar are not added. This indicates that the sodium and sugar naturally occur in the product, indicating that it is ok for consumption by you on this diet.

Things you *can* **have** during the six week period.

Fructose (found in Health Store of diabetic section
        of grocer)

Mrs. Dash or McCormick's all natural Salt free spice substitute

Soy milk or rice milk

Chicken (boneless and skinless)

Turkey (ground or fresh, but not Butterball)

Whole Wheat, Spinach, Barley, or any whole grain pasta or noodles

Whole grain, or whole wheat rice

Couscus

Water

100% organic Fruit Juice from health food store

Frozen vegetables only

Honey

Sweet potatoes or yams

The above items can be used during this six week period. The following recipes can be rotated and used for the entire six weeks. I have given several options for breakfast for instance labels under 1st day breakfast, or Sunday. You could use one of the choices for this week and another one of the choices for next week. First I am going to give you a copy of the first two pages of any program I recommend to any of my clients. They all get it, and they all orally agree to these pages before I will explain the program to them. It says:

"In the next few pages, you will find a taylor made program designed for your specific needs. If you follow the recommendations, you will get results, if you do not, you will not get results. A 50 or 75% effort on a healthy diet can be just as detrimental as a junk food diet, it is essential that the recommendations be followed promptly and precisely.

If you do, however, follow the recommendations for your program, more energy, established good health will appear, and health problems that seemed to taunt you will disappear.

Almost 90% of all health problems can be directly related back to nutrition and ultimately what is put into your mouth. Knowing this, it only stands to reason that almost 90% of all ailments can be helped by nutrition alone.

Any questions you might have, as well as long distance help, is at your disposal. Please feel free to call me at any time if you have any questions.

We are partners on this quest, and please remember, have fun, and enjoy permanent weight loss and permanent good health".

This is a copy everyone gets. I regret that I

cannot be available for the thousands who read this books, but I do still feel that if you do read these recommendations, we are all on this quest together. I also feel that there is no distance in the Spirit, and when you receive this book, whether from a friend, or a bookstore, you will receive an extra bonus with it. You will receive my continual prayers that God will literally change your life through the information contained within, and that somehow, you will become closer to our Lord Jesus Christ.

The following is a list of recipe's you can use, as well as your own when sticking to the do's and do not's listed above:

Breakfast choices

One bowl of either;

Shredded Wheat

Cream of Wheat

Wheat Germ

Regular (not instant) Oatmeal
Two slices whole wheat bread with All-fruit spread or honey

Honey dew melon, up to 16 Oz.

Cantaloupe up to 16 Oz.
Your favorite fruit, plum, apple, banana, etc., can be added to each of the above selections

One 8 Oz Glass of either;

100% Organic fruit juice

Vegetable drink made in juicer (If you do this, add an apple or two for taste)

Fruit drink made in juicer

Water- no limit

Keep in mind, I want you to choose from one of the above each day. There are five choices, if you choose a different one each day, you will not get bored. Also when you sweeten your foods, use either fructose or honey. Another helpful suggestion may be to add slices of your favorite fruit to the cereal. Also keep in mind, if you do not get full because of the amount you are used to eating, that is a good thing. We want to be in control of our bodies, and not let our bodies dictate our actions. Most people, however, have the opposite reaction usually saying that they cannot eat all I recommend them to.

Morning snack

Any vegetable or fruit such as:

Two celery stalks

Carrot

Apple

Orange

Banana

It is vital that you keep your eliminatory organs going in order to continue to clean your system out, therefore, you must keep the digestive system busy. The two snacks daily are a vital part of the six week cleansing process.

Lunch selections

Turkey sandwich on whole wheat bread (mustard only on bread @ add veggies to sandwich)

Bowl of homemade soup (recipe page after menu's)

Salad with broiled chicken mixed
with homemade Italian dressing

Chicken sandwich

Tuna Fish (in water only) sandwich

MUST! drink two glassed of water with lunch

    The above sandwiches can be eaten by themselves or in conjunction with a bowl of soup, depending on how hungry you are. Load the sandwich up, and for seasoning, use Mrs. Dash, McCormick's listed above, or just plain black pepper.

Afternoon Snack

Same as morning snack. More suggestions:

Small box of raisins

Grapes

Prunes

Pineapple

Peach

Tangerine

You get the picture, and again I cannot emphasize the importance of these snacks.

Evening meal

Ground turkey Hamburger on Whole Wheat bread

Bar-b-que chicken or turkey leg

Steamed vegetables

Garlic and Herb baked chicken
Large salad with turkey or chicken added

Chicken and whole wheat rice stir fry

Ground turkey stew

Morning Star meatless stew

Turkey Meat Loaf

Chicken and Brown Rice Soup

Chicken or Turkey Stew

Baked Fish

Turkey or Zucchini Casserole

At least one Glass of Water

100% Organic Fruit Juice (if possible from a juicer)

Please keep in mind that for this evening meal, you are allowed to eat a salad before the main course. Also you may find it helpful if you would make a soy protein shake with soy milk and soy protein mix about 15 to 30 minutes before your meal. This serves to fill you up and keeps you from eating such a large portion. It is also very good for you in that vegetable protein does not have the negative effect that animal protein does.

Now we will go into how to create your favorite meals for your nutritional change after your original six week cleansing period. Firstly, you can add to the list of things that you can eat after the initial six week period such as:

Lean Beef or pork (organic if possible) only three meals per week *

Corn only three meals per week *

I can't believe it's not butter (spray only, tub has

different ingredients *

Egg substitutes

Fried or baked potatoes (fry in olive or Canola oil only) twice weekly

Eggs (free range only)   four weekly

Hash browns (fried in olive or Canola oil only) once weekly

Buck Wheat pancakes (eat with honey or unsulphured molasses only)

Now, lets learn how to create our own menu from our favorite meals. Let's begin by looking at two different recipes for spaghetti. The first (one on the left) will be a regular recipe. The second (one on the right) will be our new recipe.

First recipe	Second recipe
1 Can spaghetti sauce	1 12 Oz can salt free tomato soup
1 LB hamburger meat	1lb morning star meatless or ground turkey
1 tbsp. Salt	1 8oz can Tomato sauce

4 Oz mushrooms	4 Oz mushrooms
1 Tsp. garlic	1tsp garlic
1 onion	1 onion
1tsp celery salt	1/4 cup celery
Spaghetti noodles	Whole Wheat noodles Noodles

Brown meat, add other Brown meatless, ingredients and add other simmer for and spices with itat least one hour simmer for 15 minutes Add 1tsp oil Boil water with 1 tbsp. butter Boil water

(I cant believe it's not butter spray)

Add noodles and boil for 15 minutes.
Rinse noodles after 15 min, serve.

Add whole grain noodles. Boil for 5 minutes, rinse noodles, serve

As you can see, *any normal recipe can be made into a recipe you can use just by substituting the original ingredients with an allowed ingredient.* The following are recipes that were on the recommendation for the menu's I suggested. After I list these, I will then give you a full and comprehensive list of ingredients and substitutions for them. In doing this, you can have the list readily available when you prepare your favorite meals just by substituting your original product with one approved on the substitution list.

Oil and vinegar salad dressing

Two or three (depending on your taste) parts olive oil to one part apple cider vinegar.
Add desired chopped vegetables. You can use any vegetables you wish. Add two tablespoons of McCormick's all herb salt free seasoning, or Mrs. Dash. Shake well.
If you wish, you can add 1/3 can of frozen pineapple juice to this recipe.

Chili
Brown one pound ground turkey, Morning Star Meatless, or Tofu. Chop onions and celery to taste and simmer with meat. Add 6 small cans no-salt tomato sauce and two cans of diced tomatoes (fresh). Add two quarts of water and three to five
tablespoons chili powder. Add 1 tablespoon of paprika and 1/2 teaspoon black pepper. Simmer for twenty minutes. That's It!

Potato Soup

Take ten medium red potatoes and cut up. Simmer onions and celery and green peppers in a 1 Tbsp olive oil and 1/8 cup water, using a 4-6 quart cooking kettle. After simmering for 5 minutes, add potatoes in kettle and fill 3/4 with water. Boil potatoes for 20 minutes at full boil, or until soft. Stir to keep from overflow. After potatoes are soft, add one half of a spray container of I can't believe it's not Butter spray, and two cups of soy milk. Add seasonings to your taste. Add one small package of frozen green peas. Brown 1 pound of ground turkey or soy protein meatless, and add to mixture. Use instant potato flakes to thicken, or corn starch and water to thicken.

Stir fry Tofu or Chicken

Get one package of Tofu or cut up chicken breasts. Stir fry in pan or wok using Olive or Canola oil. Add desired frozen vegetables and season to taste. Stir fry until vegetables and meat are hot, thawed and ready to eat. Put over brown, whole grain rice.

Turkey Meat Loaf

Brown one pound of Ground Turkey or meatless product. Add one carton egg beaters. Ad 1/4 cup while wheat flour. Add desired chopped vegetables to mixture. Mold to shape. Make groove in top of meat loaf. Add one can of no salt tomato sauce. Make aluminum foil oven in pan and put meat into it. Add one package of frozen mixed vegetables around outside of meat. Pre-heat oven to 375 degrees and cook for one hour and fifteen minutes.

Barbecue sauce

Take one teaspoon no salt Worcestershire sauce. One small can tomato sauce, one tbsp. mustard and a few drops of hickory flavoring. There you go!

The above recipes are only suggestions. As I indicated to you before, you can make your favorite meals, or any meal found in any cookbook. You only have to substitute allowed ingredients for the ones you are not allowed to have. Listed below is the substitution list I promised, the earlier list was partial,
but the following is a more complete list and included for your shopping convenience and reference:

Sugar	Fructose or Honey
Salt	McCormick's Salt free Mrs. Dash
Eggs	Egg Substitutes
Milk	Soy or rice milk
Sour Cream weekly only)	Cottage Cheese (twice
Cheese	Soy Cheese
Red Meat	(Three meals Only weekly)
Pork	(Three meals Only weekly)
Spaghetti Noodles	Whole grain, Soy, barley, Whole wheat Noodles

Rice	Whole grain Brown rice
Coffee	Decaf Coffee
Soda	Organic fruit Juice 100%
Tea	Decaf Tea
Hamburgers	Morning star Meatless patties
Sausage	Morning star Meatless Saus.
Bacon	Morning star Meatless Bacon
Hot Dogs	Morning star hot Meatless Dogs

Bread WhRemember, try to use only frozen vegetables when possible. When using canned sauces, only use salt free sauces. Check the ingredients list on canned products to make sure no salt or sugar is added. That's it, isn't that easy? With the items listed, you should be able to create any recipe you had previously. The taste, however, may be different, and you must have patience.

The vitamin portion of the six week program listed first in this chapter is usually the same for most people. The only exception being if physical problems need a modification of the program. The general daily vitamin regimen listed first in the vitamin section of this book is the same recommended for the 6 week cleansing program, only the dosage is three times daily instead of once daily. For six weeks, the recommended dosages are taken three times daily, and after the initial six weeks, it goes down to once daily in the morning.

The Herbal part of the six week period is simple. There is none! Herbs should only recommended for people going throughout the program after someone has talked to that person in length. Though I have made recommended herbs earlier in the book, they were recommended for specific cases. In this case, as I have stated many times, every person has different needs, and to assume yours without a proper initial consultation would be totally inappropriate.

In conclusion, you have been armed with an arsenal of decisions and choices to be made by you. You have recipes, and substitution lists that will allow you to create many different meals using your imagination. In doing this, you can have fun, and at the same time cleanse the Temple of God. Remember, this is a commandment of his, and we need to cut the enemies plan off now, before it's too late.

"Your Spirit Temple"

One last point I thing that merit's mentioning is your mental and spiritual wellbeing and their effect on your physical body. Any type of Doctor from a Psychologist or Psychiatrist, to a Biologist or Podiatrist will tell you that the mental health of a person has a direct relation to the bodies ability to exist. The bodies many mazes of hormones, chemicals, or organs will not operate to it's full potential if a person's mental wellbeing is not what it should be.

I can tell you one thing, all of the psychological problems in the world could be corrected by my doctor. His name is Doctor Jesus. He can correct the problem no matter how difficult it is. Despite your physical condition, all of the vitamins, herbs, and diets in the world cannot help you if your mental state is disrupted, and to state a fact, any person on the face of the earth cannot have a proper mental state if he/she does not have a proper relationship with Jesus Christ. I have been around the world twice, seen many people searching and unhappy. I have had a chief Psychiatrist break down in tears in front of me admitting that he had been contemplating suicide. I have taken in drifters to my home who think themselves wise, only to find out that throughout their lives, the only thing they had really been searching for is a personal relationship with Jesus Christ.

If you do not know Jesus Christ as your savior, he is only a prayer away. If you close your eyes and say to him, "Jesus, I know I am a sinner. I confess with my mouth my sins, and ask you to come into my life, and be the Lord of my life". If you say these words, please find a local church who believes in the miracles of our Lord and Savior Jesus Christ. Though I personally do not believe in denominations, find a church who believes Jesus Christ is the son of God, and the only way to heaven is to be born again, to confess with your mouth that he is God, that he has died and rose from the dead, and lives today in our hearts, and most importantly that Jesus Christ is the only way to heaven. If you find a church with these core values, you are one the right track.

Romans: 10:9 "That if thou shalt confess with thy mouth the Lord Jesus, and shalt believe in thine heart that God hath raised him from the dead, thou shalt be saved."

CONCLUSION!

Though this book covers the general requirements and recommendations of many things, it by no means goes into the intricate changes that have to be made in the normal course of creating a program for an individual. Many times diets will have to be modified during the course of the initial six week period, as well as supplementation and herbal modifications. Also after the initial six week period, depending on the person, many in depth adjustment may be needed, calories may need to be counted as well as protein grams, fat grams, polyunsaturated fats, monounsaturated fats. Sodium, cholesterol, fiber and carbohydrates many times must be modified for an individual. This book, however, is an anointed revelation from the Lord, and as a guide for Christians, I have not found any book with the same information.

Please realize that the programs that have been discussed within these pages by no means can substitute for proper medical help, and cannot replace the care of a health care professional. As I explained earlier, each individual is different and prayer and hearing the Lord Jesus Christ and the path he chooses for you in healing is always the first step towards living a long and healthy life.

I hope you have enjoyed the message, and I pray a blessing on all who read the words within, and pray that God will honor your willingness to head the spiritual message contained within. In finality, God Bless you and keep you.

With love in Christ, Dr. Neal.

To schedule a speaking engagement at your church or business, or to schedule a book signing please contact Dr. Schiesske at

DrLean@Yahoo.com